SYNTHETIC SUBSTRATES IN CLINICAL BLOOD COAGULATION ASSAYS

DEVELOPMENTS IN HEMATOLOGY

VOLUME 1

SYNTHETIC SUBSTRATES IN CLINICAL BLOOD COAGULATION ASSAYS

edited by

H.R. LIJNEN, D. COLLEN, M. VERSTRAETE

Center for Thrombosis and Vascular Research,
Department of Medical Research, University of Leuven

1980

MARTINUS NIJHOFF PUBLISHERS
THE HAGUE / BOSTON / LONDON

Distributors:

for the United States and Canada

Kluwer Boston, Inc.
190 Old Derby Street
Hingham, MA 02043
USA

for all other countries

Kluwer Academic Publishers Group
Distribution Center
P.O. Box 322
3300 AH Dordrecht
The Netherlands

ISBN-13: 978-94-009-8912-2 e-ISBN-13: 978-94-009-8910-8
DOI: 10.1007/978-94-009-8910-8

This conference was made possible by a grant from the
Nationaal Fonds voor Wetenschappelijk Onderzoek, Brussels;
Katholieke Universiteit Leuven;
KabiVitrum bv, Amsterdam

PREFACE

This book contains the proceedings of a symposium on the use of synthetic substrates in clinical blood coagulation assays, which was held at the University of Leuven, Belgium, on March 1st, 1980. This meeting was organized in order to exchange and discuss recent developments and applications in this field.

Advantages and disadvantages of synthetic substrates are discussed, while expert workers report on their practical experience with the use of chromogenic substrates in routine assays for blood coagulation and fibrinolysis. The indications when to perform antithrombin III, α_2- antiplasmin, factor X and factor II determinations are discussed. For each of the determinations a critical evaluation of the chromogenic assay as compared to the classical assay is presented. The clinical relevance of these assays for anticoagulated and cirrhotic patients, detection of vitamin K deficiency, monitoring heparin therapy and the fibrinolytic system are discussed. Recent developments in the use of fluorogenic substrates for the assay of low concentrations of fibrinolytic activators are presented.

Taking into account all practical, medical and economical considerations an answer is prepared to the question "Are synthetic substrates to be recommended for routine use?".

To make this symposium useful, rapid publication of the proceedings has been undertaken.

We are grateful to the participants in this meeting for their co-operation and for their willingness to provide manuscripts of their presentations. The manuscripts provided by C. Kluft and H.H.D.M. Van Vliet were presented previously at the first Amstol Symposium, Amsterdam 1978, and were updated for this publication.

H.R. LIJNEN
D. COLLEN
M. VERSTRAETE

Leuven, Belgium, June 25, 1980.

CONTRIBUTORS AND PARTICIPANTS

Dr. U. Abildgaard, Medical Department A, Aker Hospital, Oslo, Norway.

Dr. G. Baele, Department of Medicine, Coagulation Laboratory, Univ. of Ghent, Ghent, Belgium.

Dr. R.M. Bertina, Hemostasis and Thrombosis Research Unit, Dept. of Medicine, University Hospital Leiden, Leiden, The Netherlands.

Dr. A.D.J. Birch, Department of Haematology, King's College Hospital Medical School, London, U.K.

Dr. C.A. Bouvier, Haemostasis Unit, Geneva University Hospital, Geneva, Switzerland.

Dr. M. Castel, Laboratoire Central d'Hématologie, Hôtel-Dieu, 75181 Paris Cédex 04, France.

Dr. B. Cazenave, Laboratoire Central d'Hématologie, Hôtel-Dieu, 75181 Paris Cédex 04, France.

Dr. D. Collen, Center for Thrombosis and Vascular Research, Department of Medical Research, University of Leuven, Leuven, Belgium.

Dr. J. Conard, Laboratoire Central d'Hématologie, Hôtel-Dieu, 75181 Paris Cédex 04, France.

Dr. R. Douenias, Laboratoire Central d'Hématologie et d'Immunologie, Hôpital Bretonneau, 75018 Paris, France.

Dr. P. Friberger, Kabi AB, Peptide Research, Mölndal, Sweden.

Dr. H.C. Hemker, Department of Biochemistry, State University of Limburg, Maastricht, The Netherlands.

Dr. H.A. Holm, Medical Department A, Aker Hospital, Oslo, Norway.

Dr. M.H. Horellou, Laboratoire Central d'Hématologie, Hôtel-Dieu, 75181 Paris Cédex 04, France.

Dr. L.H. Kahlé, Department of Hematology, Wilhelmina Hospital, Amsterdam, The Netherlands.

Dr. V.V. Kakkar, Thrombosis Research Unit, King's College Hospital Medical School, London, U.K.

Dr. C. Kluft, Gaubius Institute, Health Research Organization TNO, Leiden, The Netherlands.

Dr. M. Knös, Kabi AB, Peptide Research, Mölndal, Sweden.

Dr. F. Laerum, Medical Department A, Aker Hospital, Oslo, Norway.

Dr. H.G. Lasch, Zentrum für Innere Medizin am Klinikum der Justus-Liebig Universität, 6300 Giessen, Germany.

Dr. H.R. Lijnen, Center for Thrombosis and Vascular Research, Department of Medical Research, University of Leuven, Leuven, Belgium.

Dr. E.A. Loeliger, Hemostasis and Thrombosis Research Unit, Department of Medicine, Univ. Hospital Leiden, Leiden, The Netherlands.

Dr. G.A. Marbet, Coagulation and Fibrinolysis Laboratory, Kantonsspital, 4031 Basel, Switzerland.

Dr. I.R. McGregor, Thrombosis Research Unit, King's College Hospital Medical School, London, U.K.

Dr. R.S. Mibashan, Department of Haematology, King's College Hospital, Medical School, London, U.K.

Dr. W. Nieuwenhuizen, Gaubius Institute, Health Research Organization TNO, Leiden, The Netherlands.

Dr. W.R.S. North, King's College Hospital Medical School and Clinical Research Centre, London, U.K.

Dr. M.M. Samama, Laboratoire Central d'Hématologie, Hôtel-Dieu, 75181 Paris Cédex 04, France.

Dr. N. Schlegel, Laboratoire Central d'Hématologie et d'Immunologie, Hôpital Bretonneau, 75018 Paris, France.

Dr. T.H. Schöndorf, Zentrum für Innere Medizin am Klinikum der Justus-Liebig Universität, 6300 Giessen, Germany.

Dr. M.F. Scully, Thrombosis Research Unit, King's College Hospital Medical School, London, U.K.

Dr. J.J. Sixma, Department of Hematology, State University Hospital, Utrecht, The Netherlands.

Dr. J.W. Ten Cate, Department of Haematology, Wilhelmina Hospital, Amsterdam, The Netherlands.

Dr. D.P. Thomas, National Institute for Biological Standards and Control, Holly Hill, Hampstead, London NW3 6RB, U.K.

Dr. J.K. Thumpston, Department of Haematology, King's College Hospital Medical School, London, U.K.

Dr. W.G. Van Aken, Central Laboratory of the Netherlands Red Cross Blood Transfusion Service, Amsterdam, The Netherlands.

Dr. H.H.D.M. Van Vliet, University Hospital Dijkzigt, Department of Hematology, Rotterdam, The Netherlands.

Dr. E.M. Van Wijk, Department of Hematology, Wilhelmina Hospital, Amsterdam, The Netherlands.

Dr. M. Verstraete, Center for Thrombosis and Vascular Research, Department of Medical Research, University of Leuven, Leuven, Belgium.

Dr. G. Wijngaards, Gaubius Institute, Health Research Organization TNO, Leiden, The Netherlands.

Dr. L. Wijnja, Laboratory of Haematology, Department of Internal Medicine, Roman Catholic Hospital, Groningen, The Netherlands.

Dr. T. Wolland, Medical Department A, Aker Hospital, Oslo, Norway.

CONTENTS

THE FIBRINOLYTIC SYSTEM

INTRODUCTION

ADVANTAGES, PITFALLS, AND SNAGS WITH CHROMOGENIC SUBSTRATES

H.C. HEMKER
Department of Biochemistry, State University of Limburg, Maastricht, The Netherlands.

Chromogenic substrates allow those interested in blood clotting and fibrinolytic enzymes to follow the activity of these enzymes continuously with the aid of a spectrophotometer. This is a major new tool in the study of these enzymes. Like any new tool, it takes some time to become acquainted with its possibilities and limitations so that we can use it optimally. This communication will stress some of the more obvious pitfalls and snags that stand in the way of an advantageous use of these substances. I will discuss the following main points :

1. The difference between bioassay and chemical assay.
2. The specificity of spectrophotometric assays.

1. BIOASSAY VERSUS CHEMICAL ASSAY

In a chemical assay there is a suitable model available for the reaction under study but in the bioassay the reaction mechanism is unknown. The titration of an unknown amount of acid with a volume of base solution of known strength is a simple example of a chemical assay. The reaction mechanism is that one molecule of acid will be neutralized by one molecule of base. An example of bioassay is the determination of a vitamin in an unknown preparation by measuring the gain in weight of deficient animals. The relation between weight and vitamin intake is complex and unknown, but on the assumption that the same amount of vitamin will cause the same increase in weight it is at least possible to compare the vitamin content of different preparations and therefore also to compare an unknown preparation with a known standard.

In the bioassay the system is a black box, the input - output characteristic of which has to be determined. Then the measurement of a certain output will allow conclusions about the input. Most coagulation assays are bioassays in this sense. The output usually is a clotting time, the standard input are known concentrations of coagulation factors in the form of dilutions of standard normal plasma. It is not true that using chromogenic substrates automatically makes a chemical assay out of these bioassays. Very often the only change upon switching to spectrophotometric methods is that now yellow colour instead of coagulation time is produced out of the same black box. Yet this use of chromogenic substrates as indicators in a bioassay does have its advantages. The clinical chemist will feel more at ease with this type of technique, it is easily automated and no specialized personnel is necessary.

On the other hand, not all clotting methods are bioassays. It has been possible to formulate a phenomenological law for the extrinsic coagulation system so that in this case at least a mathematical model is available (1). Anyhow, it is not true that the use of chromogenic substrates automatically brings coagulation factor estimations in the realm of chemical assays and therefore increases reliability and accuracy. Even if the "black-box-type-of-assay" is developed for the estimation of a given coagulation factor, a basic knowledge of enzyme kinetics and a thorough knowledge of the kinetic constants involved is required. The reader is referred to standard texts on enzyme kinetics for an introduction to this subject (2,3).

One should be aware of the fact that the relation between substrate concentration and reaction velocity is hyperbolic (Fig. 1) and that the parameters of this hyperbola are given by the two parameters K_m and V_{max} . K_m is the concentration at which half maximal reaction velocity is achieved; V_{max} is the maximal reaction velocity obtained at infinite substrate concentration. This V_{max} is proportional to the enzyme concentration and k_{cat} is the proportionality constant, i.e. $V_{max} = k_{cat}\,E$.

The hyperbolic relationship between substrate concentration and reaction velocity is given by the following formula :

$$v = \frac{k_{cat} E\ S}{K_m + S}$$

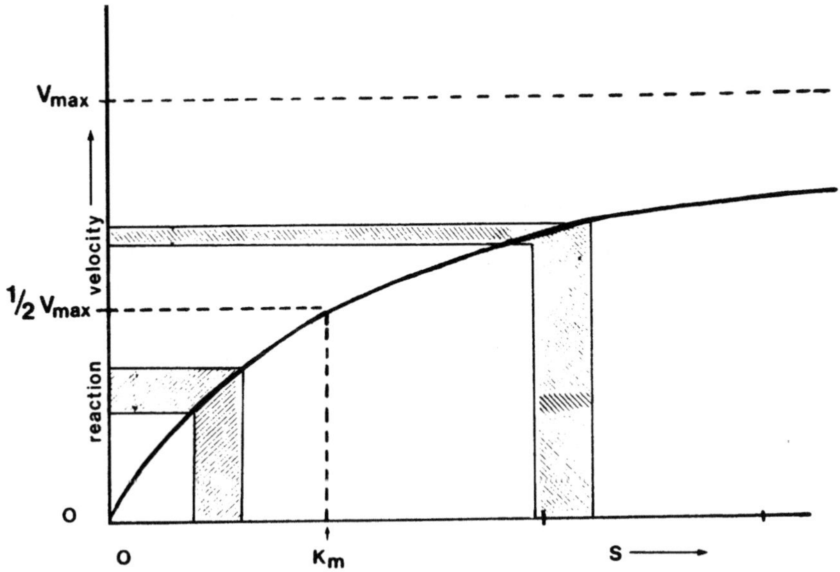

FIGURE 1. Dependence of reaction velocity on substrate consumption. A decrease in substrate concentration will cause a small decrease of reaction velocity at high substrate concentrations but a large one at low substrate concentrations.

This formula holds for initial reaction rates only, i.e. it is only valid when decrease in substrate concentration by the action of the enzyme will not appreciably decrease the reaction rate. This explains why the concentration of substrate should be well above K_m if one wants to estimate enzyme concentration (E) from the measurement of reaction velocities (v). Also it is evident that knowledge of both K_m and k_{cat} are essential in designing as well as in evaluating a test with chromogenic substrates.

It will be clear that tests in which the amount of substrate becomes rate limiting (e.g. 4) are less suitable. Also it is very often seen that reaction conditions under which the kinetic constants have been measured are not identical to those of the test in which they are used (sometimes the conditions are not specified). As the constants can vary grossly with pH, temperature and ionic strength, this is to be avoided by all means.

In this context, it may be useful to stress that if possible at least an attempt should be made to analyze data in terms of known reaction mechanisms. In coagulation often a portion of the cascade can be isolated so that the operative mechanism is of the type :

$$P \xrightarrow{U} E \quad S \xrightarrow{E} C$$

where U is the unknown enzyme to be estimated, P is a proenzyme present in excess, converted into an active enzyme E. E then converts the chromogenic substrate S into a coloured product. It is evident that if the production of E is linear in time, the production of C will be parabolical. By plotting C against t^2 (t=time), such parabolas can be conveniently analyzed (5). Yet one sees them sometimes interpreted in terms of a lag time and a subsequent linear reaction rate (6). Obviously, much information is lost in this way and interpretation of the data will be made difficult.

2. SPECIFICITY OF SPECTROPHOTOMETRIC ASSAYS

Coagulation proteases are very specific for their natural substrates and if chromogenic substrates are to be of any use, they have to show the same type of specificity. This, however, is an inherent impossibility with relatively small substrates because the natural specificity is a function of the size of the substrate. The active centre of an activated clotting protease (f II_a, X_a, VII_a, IX_a, XI_a, XII_a) breaks an amide bond in a way that is perfectly similar to that of all other serine proteases (trypsin, elastase etc.). The fact that it does break such bonds only in a limited number of susceptible proteins and at specified loci is because the activated factor and its substrate show many more interactions than the single one between active site and vulnerable site. In this way it is possible for them to fit closely together in one or few specific manner(s) and in this way the active site will meet and can act upon one (or two) specific bonds only. The number of possible interacting sites that enables such a close fit is directly related to the size of the molecule and so the size determines the specificity. A small molecule like tosyl arginine methyl ester is split by almost all serine proteases. Splitting off of the fibrinopeptides A and B in fibrinogen is done by thrombin only.

A chromogenic substrate like S-2238 or chromozym TH sufficiently mimics fibrinogen in order to be conveniently split by thrombin, nevertheless, it will be split by several other activated clotting factors to some extent.

Therefore, it is of paramount importance to ensure that these possible contributions to substrate splitting do not actually disturb the assay. Various procedures such as the presence of inhibitors, the selection of activation conditions or of the reaction circumstances (pH, ion species present, ionic strength) can ensure a more or less specific reaction.

The next drawback of chromogenic substrates is that amidase activity is not necessarily the same as biological activity. Two examples will suffice. Thrombin has an esterase (and hence amidase) activity that is not parallel to its capability to split fibrinogen. In fact, upon denaturation a thrombin molecule will first loose its clotting potency and only afterwards its esterase activity will be lost. In terms of molecular interactions this is not surprising because as already mentioned when we discussed specificity, more molecular determinants are necessary for biological functions than for catalytic activity per se. This discrepancy is not likely to be a serious problem with freshly generated thrombin but it does play a disturbing role in purified preparations such as those used for a thrombin standard (7).

A second example is readily found in the abnormal prothrombin present in the blood during oral anticoagulation or vitamin K deficiency. This protein that we called Protein Induced by Vitamin K Absence or Antagonists (PIVKA) is identical to normal prothrombin but for the absence of γ-COOH-glutamic acid residues in its N-terminal end (8). As these groups serve to anchor the protein to a phospholipid surface, the physiological activation that occurs at such a surface is seriously impaired. Other types of activation such as those by Echis Carinatus venom or staphylocoagulase do generate protease activity as readily from PIVKA-II as from normal factor II. A factor II estimation using one of these activators and a substrate specific for thrombin would therefore give erroneous results in cases of anticoagulant therapy but not in cases of cirrhosis of the liver or with standard dilutions of normal plasma.

A third point to be mentioned is competition between chromogenic substrates and between artificial and normal substrates. One example will serve as an illustration : when one tries to estimate thrombin generation in a plasma sample by continuous measurement of the conversion of a chromogenic substrate specific for thrombin, can one expect that the results do represent thrombin generation in that sample as if no chromogenic substrate were present? Indeed, at every moment the rate of colour production will be a good estimate of the amount of free thrombin available. The conversion of the substrate by factor X_a and other clotting proteases can safely be disregarded because

a. their amount is small compared to that of thrombin, and
b. they will split the chromogenic substrate less efficiently than thrombin does.

This, however, does not automatically imply that the added substrate will not react with factor X_a. In fact, the binding of the substrate to factor X_a can be appreciable (i.e. when K_m is relatively small) but the splitting can be slow (k_{cat} small). In that case the substrate will act as an efficient inhibitor of factor X_a and prothrombin conversion will be slower in the presence of the substrate than in its absence.

I conclude that chromogenic substrates can be very useful tools indeed, but that their application must be backed by a thorough knowledge of the properties of the system under study, some knowledge of enzyme kinetics and lots of common sense.

REFERENCES

1. Hemker HC, Vermeer C, and Govers-Riemslag JWP. 1977. Kinetic aspects of the interaction of blood clotting enzymes. VII. The relation between clotting time and prothrombin concentration. Thrombos. Haemostas. 37, 81-85.
2. Dixon M and Webb E. 1957. Enzymes. Longmans, Green and Co., London.
3. Fersht A. 1977. Enzyme structure and mechanism. W.H. Freeman and Co. Reading, San Francisco.
4. Sandberg H and Andersson D. 1979. A highly sensitive assay of platelet factor 3 using a chromogenic substrate. Thrombos.Res. 14, 113-124.
5. Kosow DP, Furie B, and Forastieri H. 1974. Activation of factor X : kinetic properties of the reaction. Thrombos.Res. 4, 219-227.
6. Suomela H, Blombäck M, and Blombäck B. 1977. The activation of factor X evaluated by using synthetic substrates. Thrombos.Res. 10, 267-281.

7. Gaffney PJ, Lord K, Brasher M, and Kirkwood TBL. 1977. Problems in the assay of thrombin using synthetic peptides as substrates. Thrombos.Res. 10, 549-556.
8. Stenflo J, Fernlund P, Egan W, and Roepstorff P. 1974. Vitamin K dependent modifications of glutamic acid residues in prothrombin Proc.Natl.Acad.Sci. 71, 2730-2733.

DISCUSSION

D. Collen : Dr. Hemker said that it is advisable to work at a concentration of substrate that is far above the K_m in order to minimize substrate changes during the reaction. However, some of the presently available chromogenic substrates have a relatively high K_m, which makes it very difficult to work above K_m. Still, if the amount of substrate which has to be converted in order to generate enough colour represents only a small amount of the substrate concentration used, this concentration will not change during the assays and there will be no practical problem.

H.C. Hemker : Yes, if one can measure initial reaction rates one need not operate far above K_m. When one uses up till about 20 percent of the initial substrate during the test, one can still apply kinetics using the method of Lee and Anderson. This method plots the mean reaction velocity over a time lapse against the mean substrate concentration which still results in a normal saturation curve (on Lineweaver-Burk plot when the inverses are used). So, there are ways around it, but in practice it is preferable if you can be above K_m.

H.R. Lijnen : Is it not so that also the V_{max} is important in these determinations because I think you should have a large V_{max} to have a fast liberation of paranitroaniline in these determinations?

H.C. Hemker : That's partly true. The efficiency of the test is given by k_{cat} over K_m and V_{max} is k_{cat} times the enzyme concentration. As I have shown, there can be situations in which K_m is relatively low and k_{cat} is also low, and then you are in trouble because in these cases the substrate will act more as an inhibitor than as a suitable substrate.

THE COAGULATION SYSTEM

THE POTENTIAL USE OF CHROMOGENIC ASSAYS IN THE ROUTINE MONITORING OF ORAL ANTICOAGULANT THERAPY

R.M. BERTINA and E.A. LOELIGER

Hemostasis and Thrombosis Research Unit, Department of Medicine, University Hospital Leiden, Rijnsburgerweg 10, 2333 AA Leiden, The Netherlands.

INTRODUCTION

The treatment of patients with oral anticoagulants proceeds in two phases. After an initial loading dose of anticoagulant the plasma concentration of the factors VII, IX, X and II decreases each according to its own half life (1-3). This is schematically illustrated in Figure 1. The factor VII activity rapidly disappears from the plasma, while the half life of factor II is about 10 times higher. After this loading

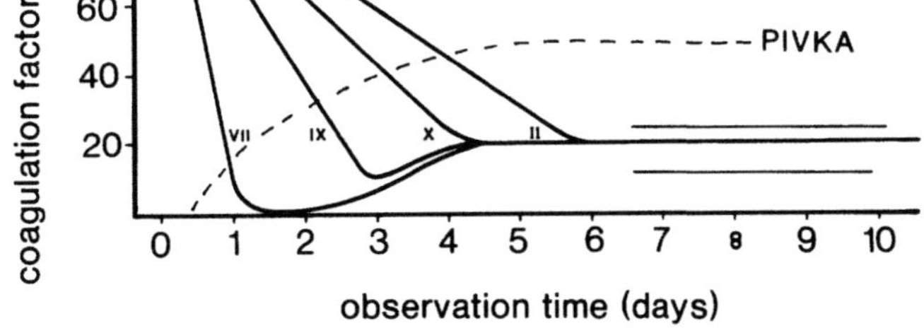

FIG. 1. Schematic representation of the procedure of oral anticoagulation.

dose, anticoagulant administration is gradually decreased until a maintenance dose is reached that results in the desired level of anticoagulation. In these so-called stabilized patients the administration of the anticoagulant is such that the percentage of inhibition of the synthesis of procoagulant factors VII, II, IX and X is virtually the same for each factor (4).

Any change in the effectiveness of the anticoagulant - as for instance introduced by interfering drugs (5-6) - will destabilize the patient until a new steady state is reached. Due to the short half life of the disappearance of factor VII(as measured after administration of a blocking dose of anticoagulant)and of the reappearance(as measured after the subsequent administration of vitamin K_1) factor VII levels will be most sensitive to changes in effectiveness of the anticoagulant.

At present the monitoring of oral anticoagulant therapy occurs by considering the result of a prothrombin time determination. The use of a factor VII sensitive thromboplastin in this determination has the advantage that it offers the possibility to prevent factor VII concentration becoming too low during the starting period of anticoagulation. A too low factor VII concentration might lead to clinical bleeding (7) and is one of the obligatory conditions for the development of haemorrhagic skin necrosis (8).

The discussion of today is focused on the question if we have available assays at present - using chromogenic substrates - that could be used in the routine monitoring of oral anticoagulant therapy. During the past 5 years the potential use of such "chromogenic" assays in the monitoring of anticoagulant therapy has been repeatedly suggested (9-13). However, at present no results have been reported detailing with a double blind prospective study which compares the use of a conventional prothrombin time with that of a "chromogenic" method.

Two types of chromogenic assays have been suggested to be promising :

1. Chromogenic assays where plasma is activated with thromboplastin and Ca^{2+} ; thrombin generation then is monitored by its activity towards a specific peptide substrate (Chromozym TH or S-2238) (9, 14-16). In fact such a method is still a prothrombin time. Only the technic of endpoint detection has been modified. Compared with a conventional prothrombin time such a method is more expensive. However, it offers different possibilities for automation which might

compensate for the extra costs of the chromogenic substrate. An apparent disadvantage of these chromogenic assays is that they still are dependent on the biological properties of thromboplastins with all the associated problems of calibration and standardization.

2. A second type of assay that has been suggested to be useful in monitoring oral anticoagulant therapy, is the spectrophotometric assay of one of the vitamin K dependent coagulation factors, especially factor II (10,17,18) and factor X (10,12,13).

During the last two years we have used spectrophotometric assays to determine factor II and factor X in the plasma of patients on oral anticoagulant therapy. Based on this experience we believe at present that these methods cannot be used for adequate monitoring of oral anticoagulation.

SPECTROPHOTOMETRIC FACTOR II AND FACTOR X ASSAY

In the spectrophotometric factor II assay prothrombin is converted into thrombin by the action of Xa in the presence of phospholipid, Ca^{2+} and factor V. The amount of thrombin formed is estimated by its amidolytic activity towards S-2238. The details of the method have been described elsewhere (18).

In the spectrophotometric factor X assay, factor X is converted into Xa by the action of Russell Viper Venom-X (RVV-X) in the presence of Ca^{2+}. The amount of Xa formed is measured by its amidolytic activity towards S-2222 or S-2337. The S-2337 was kindly made available by Kabi (Stockholm). Figure 2 shows that there is a linear relationship between the formed amidolytic activity and the plasma factor X concentration. The latter was varied by diluting pooled normal plasma in human factor X deficient plasma. We like to emphasize that all assays that use RVV-X as an activator of procoagulant factor X have to be checked with respect to the behaviour of acarboxy-factor X (PIVKA X) in the assay. Although the rate of activation of acarboxy-X by RVV-X might be relatively slow when compared with that of procoagulant factor X (19) its contribution to the total amidolytic activity might be quite significant due to the required presence of a large excess of RVV-X.

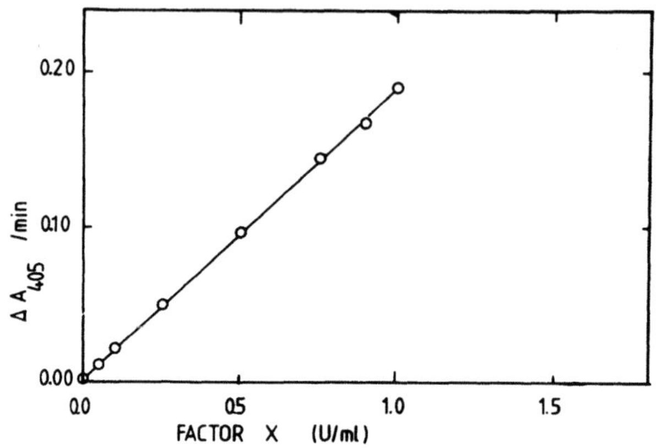

FIG. 2. Calibration curve for the spectrophotometric factor X assay. To 0.5 ml buffer (0.05 M Tris-imidazole, 0.435 M NaCl; polybrene[R], 36 µg/ml; pH 8.3) is added 0.02 ml plasma and 0.2 ml of a solution containing 0.05 M $CaCl_2$ and RVV-X (30 µg/ml); after 90 sec incubation at 37°C, 0.20 ml S-2337 solution (1.5 mM) is added; the initial rate of p-nitroaniline formation is recorded at 405 nm.

CAN THESE CHROMOGENIC ASSAYS ADEQUATELY MONITOR THE INITIAL REACTION OF THE PATIENT TO THE ANTICOAGULANT?

In Figure 3A a comparison is made between factor II and factor VII levels in the plasma of a number of patients that started oral anticoagulation less than two weeks before sampling. It is obvious that there is no correlation between factor VII and factor II levels in these patients. Factor VII concentrations of less than 0.05 U/ml can be found at factor II concentrations ranging from 0.15 U/ml to 0.50 U/ml. Figure 3B demonstrates that in plasma of patients treated for more than 6 months a good correlation exists between the concentration of factor VII and factor II. It has been suggested that factor X - because of its shorter half life - might be a better indicator for "overshooting" during the first days of treatment than factor II. Therefore plasmas with low factor VII concentration and different factor II concentrations were selected. In these samples factor X was estimated with the spectrophotometric assay (Table 1). The results show that in general the factor X concentration is slightly lower than the factor II concentration but much higher than that of factor VII.

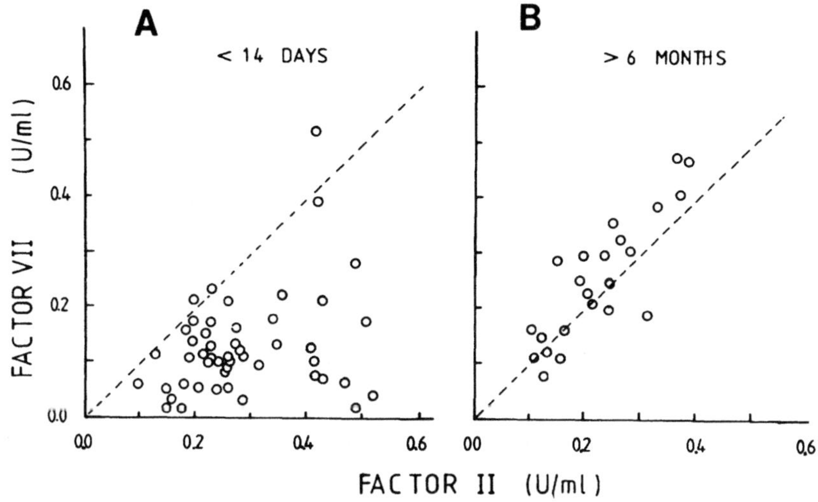

FIG. 3. Factor II and VII levels in the plasmas of patients treated with oral anticoagulants for < 14 days (A) or > 6 months (B).

TABLE 1.

Plasma levels of vitamin K dependent coagulation factors during short-term treatment with oral anticoagulants.

TT (sec)	FII (U/ml)	FX (U/ml)	FVII (U/ml)
103	0.42	0.30	0.07
134	0.18	0.18	0.06
116	0.26	0.20	0.08
94	0.27	0.28	0.08
101	0.42	0.30	0.10
184	0.18	0.16	0.01
212	0.15	0.15	0.05
139	0.29	0.22	0.03
174	0.21	0.17	0.05
146	0.26	0.22	0.05
135	0.31	0.28	0.09
116	0.34	0.28	0.17

It appears then that the use of a spectrophotometric factor X assay during the first days of anticoagulation has the same limitations as the factor II assay : it does not reflect the reaction of factor VII on the initial loading dose. So, by using such assays during the starting period, the patient control is insufficiently safe.

CAN SPECTROPHOTOMETRIC FACTOR II OR FACTOR X ASSAYS BE USED FOR ADEQUATE MONITORING OF PATIENTS STABILIZED ON ORAL ANTI-COAGULANTS?

The problem concealed in this question is, what is adequate monitoring? In practice the clinician tries to anticoagulate a patient in such a way that the prothrombin time will be prolonged with a factor that has been established empirically for a particular group of patients. The Dutch Federation of Thrombosis Services recommends prolongation ratios between 2 and 5 in terms of proposed ICRs (International Calibrated Ratio). When this ratio is lower then 2 anticoagulation is considered insufficiently effective not only for the prophylaxis of arterial thrombosis but also for the prophylaxis of venous thrombosis. When the prolongation ratio is higher than 5 the risk for bleeding disorders is high. In Britain prolongation ratios between 2 and 4 are considered as optimal. In our opinion an adequate monitoring of stabilized patients requires that the test method can indicate small changes in coagulability within the range of optimal anticoagulation. This means that there should be sufficient correlation between factor II or factor X concentration and the prothrombin time <u>within</u> the region that is considered optimal for anticoagulant treatment.

On the plasma of 53 patients - that were included in the Leiden contribution to an international calibration study of reference thromboplastins - the following determinations and assays were performed : prothrombin times with the reference thromboplastins 67/40 (human combined), 70/178 (rabbit) and 68/434 (bovine combined) factor II and factor X (spectrophotometrically). It should be noted that for all patients it was checked that the blood sample was drawn during a period of stable anticoagulation.

The results were expressed as the following ratios :

a) For the prothrombin times a prolongation ratio was calculated from the actual prothrombin time and the mean prothrombin time in a group of 20 healthy individuals : i.e. $\frac{PT}{PT_{normal}}$.

b) For factor II and factor X the ratios were calculated by which the concentration of the factor was decreased when compared with pooled normal plasma : i.e. 1.0/FX(II). We choose this particular ratio because it is known that there is an inverse relationship between the concentration of vitamin K dependent factors and the prothrombin time.

In the next figures the prolongation ratio obtained with 67/40 was plotted on the X-axis, because this thromboplastin has been accepted by the WHO in 1977 as the reference thromboplastin for oral anticoagulation (WHO, technical report, 1977) (20).

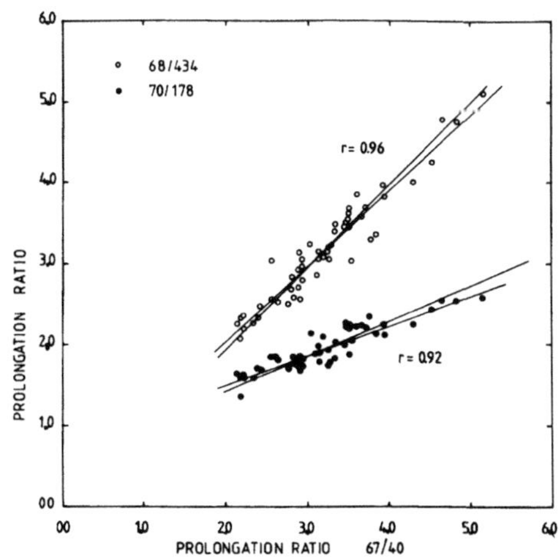

FIG. 4. Correlation between prolongation ratios obtained with 3 different thromboplastins.

Figure 4 shows that there is a good correlation between the prolongation ratios obtained with the 3 types of thromboplastin.

Figure 5 shows the correlation between 1.0/FII and the prolongation ratio obtained with 67/40; between ratios of 2 and 5 the coefficient of correlation is 0.8, while this coefficient is 0.6 when only points between ratios 2 and 4 are considered.

Figure 6 shows the correlation between 1.0/FX and the prolongation ratio. It is evident that the correlation is not good (r = 0.47); this is partly caused by the fact that at increasing prolongation

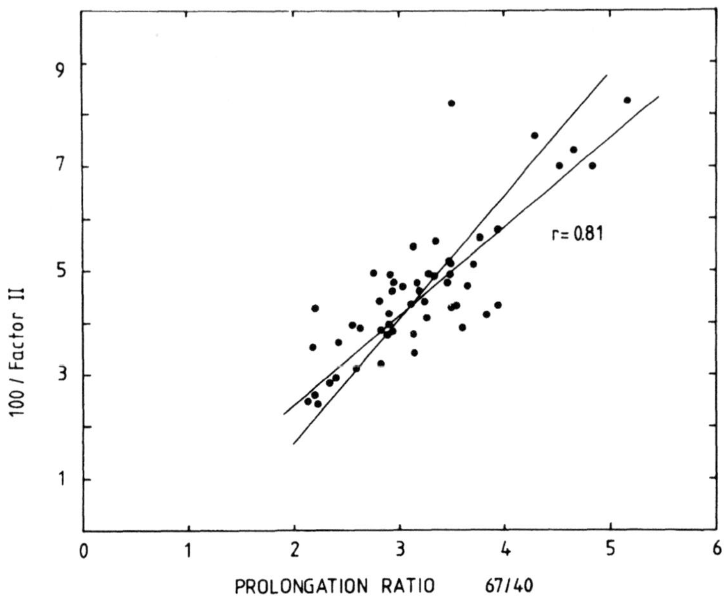

FIG. 5. Correlation between 1/FII and the prolongation ratio obtained with 67/40.

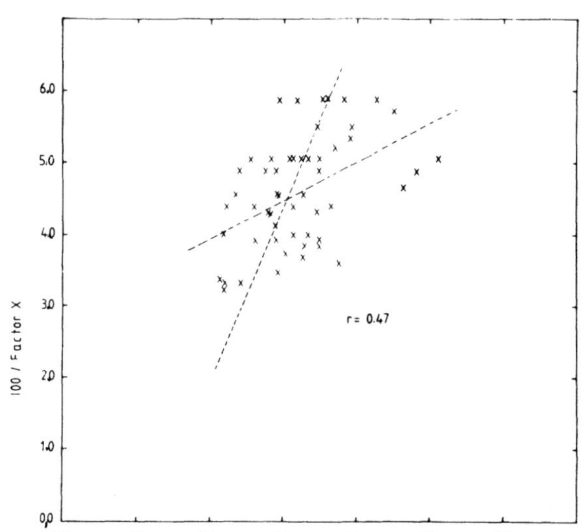

FIG. 6. Correlation between 1/FX and the prolongation ratio obtained with 67/40.

ratios the decrease of factor X is much less than for instance the decrease of factor II. This might be due to the contribution of small amounts of acarboxy-factor X in the spectrophotometric factor X assay.

Figures 7 and 8 show the data of Figures 5 and 6, plotted in another way.

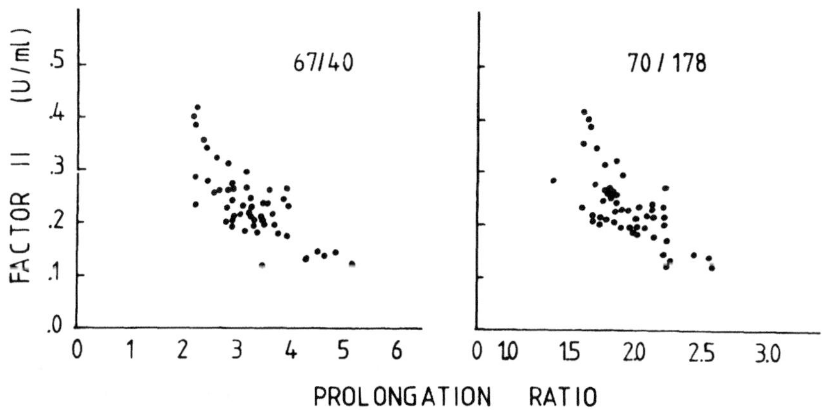

FIG. 7. Factor II as function of the prolongation ratio obtained with 67/40 or 70/178.

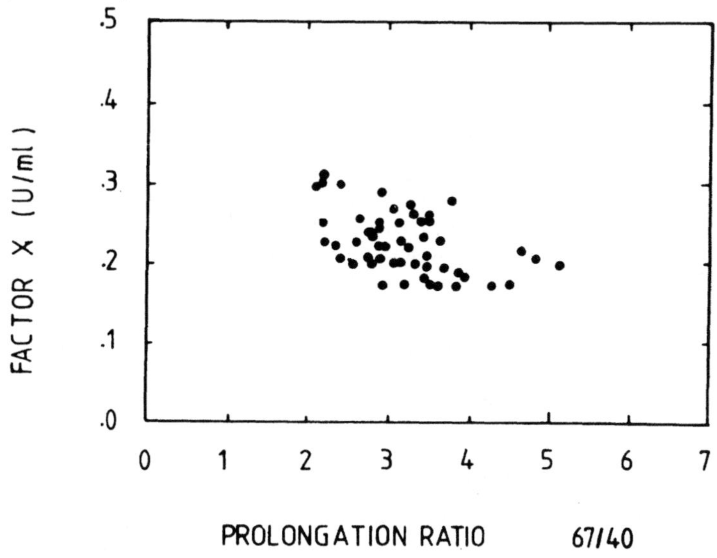

FIG. 8. Factor X as function of the prolongation ratio obtained with 67/40.

Careful consideration of these results indicates that on the base of results of a factor II or factor X assay it is impossible to make a justified decision if a particular patient is in the upper region or in the lower region of the optimal therapeutical range. Such a situation is not compatible with adequate control of the safety of the patient.

ACKNOWLEDGEMENTS

We are grateful to the National Institute for Biological Standards and Control, London, for supplying the International Reference Preparations of thromboplastin.

REFERENCES

1. Hellemans J, Vorlat M, and Verstraete M. 1963. Survival time of prothrombin and factors VII, IX and X after completely synthesis blocking doses of coumarin derivatives. Brit.J.Haemat. 9, 506-512.
2. Hjort PF, Egeberg O, and Mikkelsen S. 1961. Turnover of prothrombin, factor VII and factor IX in a patient with haemophilia A. Scand.J.Clin.Lab.Invest. 13, 668-672.
3. Kazmier FJ, Spittell JA, Thompson JJ, and Owen CA. 1965. Effect of oral anticoagulants on factors VII, IX, X and II. Arch.Intern. Med. 115, 667-673.
4. Loeliger EA, Esch B van der, Mattern MJ, and Brabander ASA den. 1963. Behaviour of factors II, VII, IX, and X during longterm treatment with coumarin. Thromb.Diath.Haemorrh. 9, 74-89.
5. Stockley IH. 1973. Interactions with oral anticoagulants - Part I. Pharmaceut.J. 210, 339-343.
6. Stockley IH. 1973. Interactions with oral anticoagulants - Part II. Pharmaceut.J. 210, 395-399.
7. Marder VJ and Shulman NR. 1964. Clinical aspects of congenital factor VII deficiency. Amer.J.Med. 37, 182-194.
8. Amstel WJ van, Boekhout-Mussert MJ, and Loeliger EA. 1978. Successful prevention of coumarin-induced hemorrhagic skin necrosis by timely administration of vitamin K_1. Blut 36, 89-93.
9. Axelsson G, Korsan-Bengtsen K, and Waldenström J. 1976. Prothrombin determination by means of a chromogenic peptide substrate. Thromb.Haemostas. 36, 517-524.
10. Bergström K and Egberg N. 1978. Determination of vitamin K sensitive coagulation factors in plasma. Studies on three methods using synthetic chromogenic substrates. Thromb.Res. 12, 531-547.
11. Kirchhof BRJ, Muller AD, Vermeer C, and Hemker HC. 1979. Control of anticoagulant therapy with a chromogenic substrate. Haemostasis 8, 1-7.

12. Lämmle B, Eichlisberger R, Hänni L, Bounameaux H, Marbet GA, and Duckert F. 1979. Kontrolle der oralen Antikoagulation : Vergleich zwischen Quick- und kolorimetrischer Factor-X-Bestimmung bei 107 Patiënten. Schweiz.Med.Wschr. 109, 1115-1119.
13. Mibashan RS, Scully MF, Birch AJ, Thumpston J, MacGregor IR, and Kakkar VV. 1979. Automated control of coumarin therapy by chromogenic factor X assay. Thromb.Haemostas. 42, 291.
14. Witt I. 1977. Determination of plasma prothrombin with chromozym TH. In : Witt I (Ed), New methods for the analysis of coagulation using chromogenic substrates. Walter De Gruyter, Berlin-New York, pp. 155-169.
15. Róka L, Koch R, and Bleyl H. 1977. Studies on the determination of prothrombin with S-2160. In : Witt I (Ed), New methods for the analysis of coagulation using chromogenic substrates. Walter De Gruyter, Berlin-New York, pp 171-179.
16. Baughan DJ and Lytwyn A. 1979. A novel chromogenic assay equivalent to the one stage prothrombin time (PT). Thromb.Haemostas. 42, 291.
17. Kirchhof BRJ, Vermeer C, and Hemker HC. 1978. The determination of prothrombin using synthetic chromogenic substrates; choice of a suitable activator. Thromb.Res. 13, 219-232.
18. Bertina RM, Marel-van Nieuwkoop W van der, Loeliger EA. 1979. Spectrophotometric assays of prothrombin in plasma of patients using oral anticoagulants. Thromb.Haemostas. 72, 1296-1305.
19. Lindhout MJ, Kop-Klaassen BHM, and Hemker HC. 1978. Activation of decarboxyfactor X by a protein from Russell's Viper Venom. Purification and partial characterization of activated decarboxyfactor X. Biochim.Biophys.Acta 533, 327-341.
20. WHO Expert Committee on Biological Standardisation. 1977. 28th Report. Technical Report Series World Health Organisation, no 610, p. 48.

DISCUSSION

H.C. Hemker : What would you expect if instead of a chromogenic assay you would use one coagulation assay to determine factor II with the use of normal thromboplastin and another with the use of Ecarin or staphylocoagulase?

R.M. Bertina : It will give the same results as the chromogenic assays.

D. Collen : Why then do you prefer chromogenic substrates above coagulation assays? Is it because of possible automation?

R.M. Bertina : I don't believe it is only because of the automation. With the chromogenic assay you only have to perform two assays; and when you are measuring levels of clotting factors you must also prepare several dilutions of standards and test samples. It takes more time.

L. Wijnja : But the normotest is a simple test in clinical use, for vitamin K deficiency. You showed that estimation of factor II is better than the conventional clotting assays, but what is your opinion for the initial use?

R.M. Bertina : We tried to select plasmas that were difficult to analyse on the base of the laboratory clotting assays; this means reduced normotest while the factor V was within the normal range. In general this would be in agreement with vitamin K deficiency. To prove vitamin deficiency in such a case vitamin K_1 is given to the patient and then the laboratory tests have to be repeated; normalisation of these tests finally proves the diagnosis of vitamin K deficiency. If we do the 2 spectrophotometric assays it is not necessary to give vitamin K_1 when no vitamin K deficiency is detected.

D. Collen : These are mild cases of vitamin K deficiency. The amount of PIVKA's you find in such patients is very low, probably of the order of 20% of the total. Does such a diagnosis have any clinical relevance?

R.M. Bertina : Each vitamin K deficiency that was suggested by the clotting test and has been proven after vitamin K administration, also was found with the chromogenic assays. But, due to the long half-time of acarboxyfactor II, there still will be some circulating acarboxyfactor II when the procoagulant factor II concentration has been largely corrected. So when the clotting tests are already corrected, you still can detect vitamin K deficiency in the chromogenic assay.

H.C. Hemker : In practice there is a rather simple way to detect vitamin K deficiency and that is to see if there is a discrepancy between normotest and thrombotest or alternatively by doing a thrombotest dilution curve. Did you investigate your patients also with this simple method?

R.M. Bertina : We did no thrombotest dilution curves and I do not agree that this test is as simple as the chromogenic assay. It still is time-consuming and in the case of liver disease it sometimes is difficult to interprete, because of the demonstration of small amounts of inhibitor (not fully carboxylated molecules).

H.C. Hemker : That will not be of practical importance because not completely carboxylated molecules will in practice act as a mixture of fully carboxylated and uncarboxylated molecules.

R.M. Bertina : Yes o.k. But the results from thrombotest dilution curves will also in the case of severe liver disease give the impression that there could be a circulating inhibitor.

H.C. Hemker : You may be right but I should have preferred to see the comparison in your test series.

AUTOMATED CONTROL OF COUMARIN THERAPY BY CHROMOGENIC FACTOR X ASSAY

M.F. SCULLY, R.S. MIBASHAN*, A.D.J. BIRCH*, J.K. THUMPSTON*, I.R. McGREGOR, W.R.S. NORTH° and V.V. KAKKAR

Thrombosis Research Unit and Department of Haematology*, King's College Hospital Medical School and Clinical Research Centre°, London.

INTRODUCTION

Therapy with coumarin anticoagulants results in reduced levels of biologically active factors II, VII, IX and X. It is usually monitored by following the prothrombin time or some similar test sensitive to deficiencies of factor II, VII and X. Such tests are not readily automated and rely on detecting fibrin clotting caused by thrombin. They are therefore affected by fibrinogen concentration and heparin as well as by coumarin induced defect. The problem of thromboplastin standardisation is also present.

The development of chromogenic peptide substrates allows specific and precise factor assays to be performed which do not have these drawbacks. In this present study the reliability of an automated factor X method for the control of the anticoagulant therapy of a series of patients stabilised on coumarin has been assessed.

MATERIALS AND METHODS

Patients

Thirty-six patients attending an out-patients clinic, already established on long term Warfarin and with a variety of previous indications for therapy were randomly selected. Samples of blood were taken at each of four consecutive monthly visits.

Plasma samples

Nine volumes of blood were added to one volume of 3.8% citrate. Plasma was prepared by centrifugation at 3000 xg for 20 min at +4° and samples stored in aliquots at -20°.

Standard curves were prepared from a normal pooled plasma which was stored in liquid nitrogen as also were two local standards prepared from anticoagulated patients.

Prothrombin Time Ratio (P.T.R.)

Values were obtained by a manual method using the Manchester Comparative Thromboplastin (Dr.L.Poller , Withington Hospital, Manchester).

Coagulant Factor X Assay

A semiautomated technique using a Schnitger and Gross coagulometer and Russells Viper Venom (RVV) in cephalin (Sigma Chemical Co) was used.

Chromogenic Factor X Assay

This was essentially according to the method of Aurell et al.(1977) (1) but was fully automated using an LKB Reaction Rate Analyser 2086 MK II linked to an LKB Kinetic Data Processor 2082. RVV was preinjected at t=60 seconds and then substrate, S2222 (KabiVitrum) at t=0. A fixed time programme was used. Samples were fed through in batches of 36 together with dilutions of plasma to prepare standard curves.

RESULTS AND DISCUSSION

Correlation of the chromogenic and coagulant assays of factor X in the coumarin affected plasmas were very closely comparable with a regression coefficient of 0.80 (Fig. 1). The fitted line did not go through the origin indicating a slightly higher apparent level of factor X as measured chromogenically to that observed by the coagulant method. This discrepancy may arise from the method of preparing standard curves by diluting normal plasma with saline (and therefore plasma inhibitors) giving slightly higher values in the direct measurement of factor Xa (chromogenic) than the indirect measurement (coagulant).

In order that warfarin dosage could be decided from either the chromogenic assay or the P.T.R. without bias the best fit regression of P.T.R. on factor X level was determined from the 144 pairs of results (Fig. 2) and the derived values substituted in the patient's record. One of us (R.S.M.) decided the appropriate dose of warfarin without knowing the patient identity or whether the P.T.R. was real

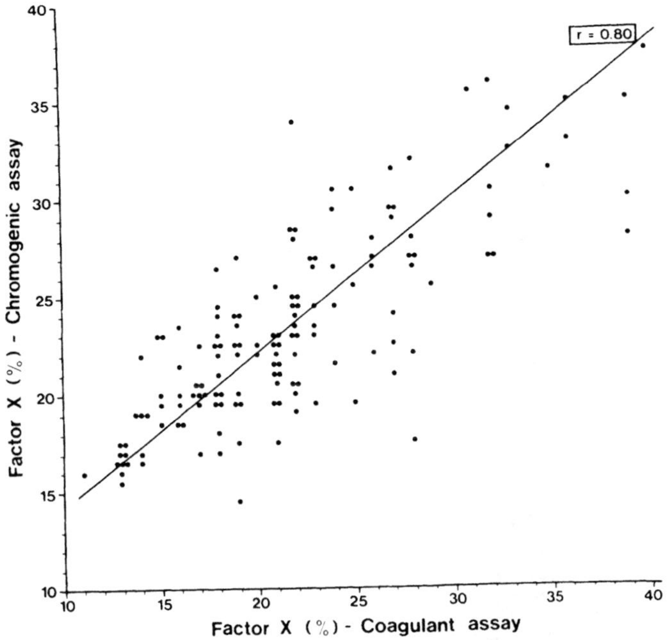

FIG. 1. Correlation of Factor X assay techniques.

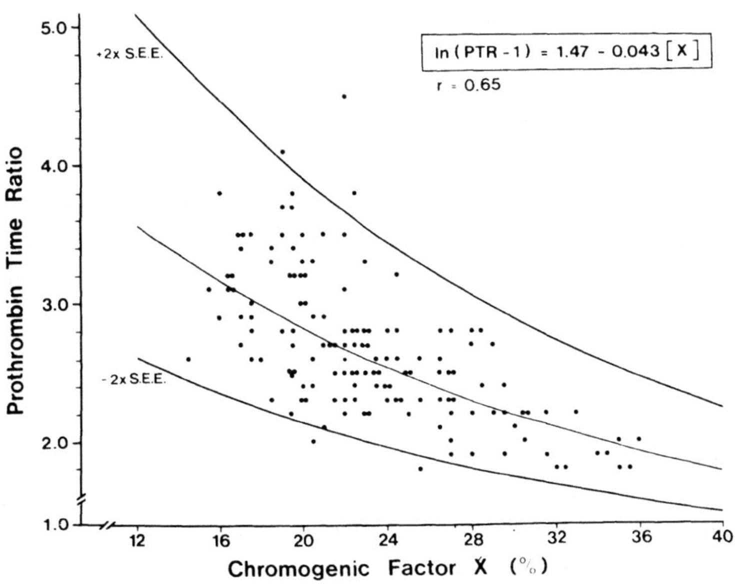

FIG. 2. Regression of P.T.R. on Factor X levels.

or derived. The plot of differences in dose shows how small the effect would have been had the patients been transferred to control with the factor X assay at each visit (Fig. 3).

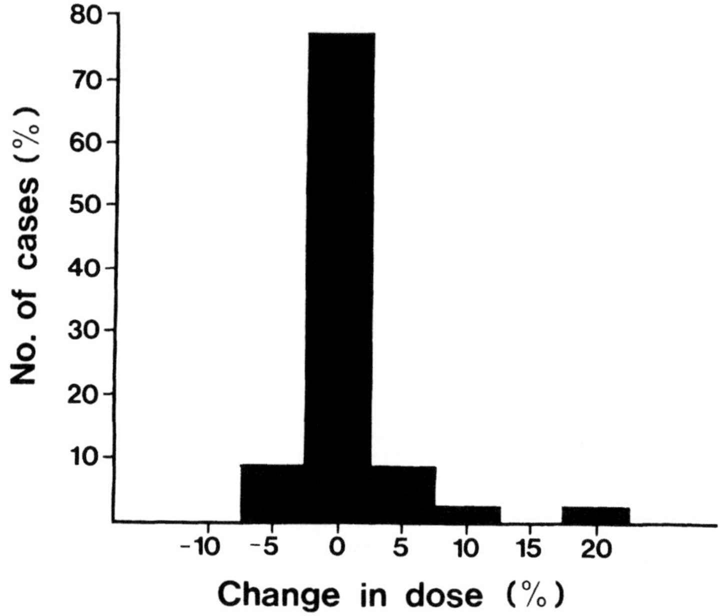

FIG. 3. Change in warfarin dose on changing from P.T.R. to Factor X levels.

Analysis of variance shows that more than half the discrepancy between P.T.R. and chromogenic factor X assay is accounted for by differences between patients ($p < 0.001$). When the results for each patient are plotted, visit by visit, the parallelism between the factor X assay and P.T.R. is most striking, but the relationship between the two tests varies from case to case (Fig. 4).

CONCLUSION

In the previously stabilised patients examined, substitution of the chromogenic factor X assay for the P.T.R. made no difference to the doses of warfarin prescribed. The relationship between factor X and P.T.R. varied unpredictably between patient, presumably as a result of differing effects of warfarin on other coumarin sensitive factors.

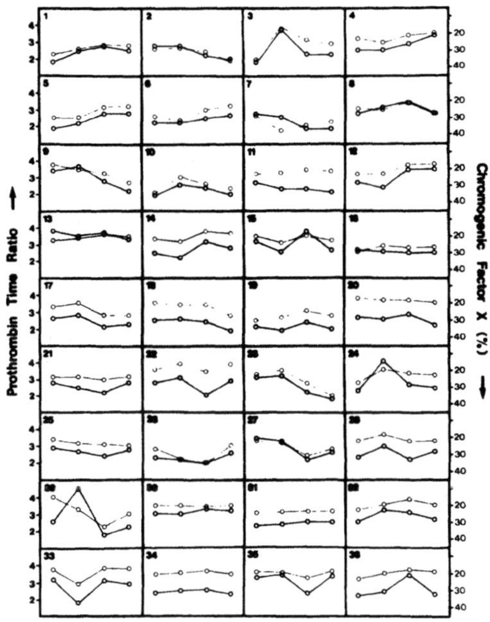

FIG. 4. Individual values for P.T.R. and Factor X in 36 patients on four occasions. Heavily barred lines are Factor X levels.

The chromogenic assay can be fully automated and offers advantages where large numbers of patients are treated. There is no clear evidence that the P.T.R. more closely reflects the inhibition of thrombosis in vivo than the factor X assay. It remains to be tested whether the lack of sensitivity to factor VII is clinically important if this method is used at the start of coumarin treatment.

REFERENCES

1. Aurell L, Friberger P, Karlsson G, and Claeson G. 1977. A new sensitive and highly specific chromogenic substrate for Factor Xa. Thrombos.Res. 11, 595-610.

DISCUSSION

P. Friberger : I would just like to comment on one item here concerning the acarboxyfactor X. We have a preparation from Dr. C. Jackson and we used it under the conditions for the assay. The activity obtained with this acarboxyfactor X was around 1% of that obtained with normal factor X. This confirms the results recently published by Lindhout. Acarboxyfactor X is activated, but at a much slower rate.

D. Collen : Apparently the correlation between the prolongation of the prothrombin time and the factor X assay with the chromogenic substrates is quite different in these three studies. Are these studies not comparing a linear change in the factor X assay with a hyperbolic or a logarithmic change in the prolongation of the prothrombin time?

H.C. Hemker : In general you'll find a linear relation between clotting time and 1/factor X in the factor X assay. This also holds for "Quick type tests" ("prothrombin times" or "thromboplastin times") because if the vitamin K dependent factors are equally low then factor X is rate limiting in these tests. Now, if you divide clotting time by the standard clotting time of normal plasma so as to obtain prothrombin time ratios, nothing changes in that linear relation. So, indeed I think you can use linear regression when you are comparing 1/coagulation factor concentration and clotting time ratios.

G.A. Marbet : We also did a comparison of factor X measured by S-2222 with the prothrombin time (human brain thromboplastin) expressed as percentage values. In 107 plasma samples of patients with stable oral anticoagulation the correlation was highly significant, $r=0.65$, $p < 0.001$. The distribution of our data looks very similar to those of the previous speakers. We have tried to prescribe oral anticoagulants according to factor X values measured by S-2222. Our therapeutic range with human brain thromboplastin of 15 to 25% corresponds to 15-28% factor X. 42 patients have been randomly allocated to one group controlled by our usual human brain thromboplastin and to another controlled by the S-2222 method. The observation period was 3 to 4 months for each patient. The number of prothrombin time values deviating from the therapeutic range during the study did not differ significantly between the two groups. Therefore we believe that monitoring of oral anticoagulation by a chromogenic substrate method might be possible without unacceptable risks for the patient. A definite answer about the value of such new methods in comparison to the prothrombin time could only be given from large clinical trials taking into account the frequency of bleeding and rethrombosis.

L.H. Kahlé : I have one comment on the comparison of these assays. In the prothrombin time you are measuring the whole cascade system from factor VII to fibrin formation, and you are comparing this with a factor X assay. Then you cannot expect a good correlation. Of course, if you compare between factor X chromogenic and factor X clotting activity you will always get a better correlation; so it is just the wrong comparison. What we did in Amsterdam was just looking at the therapeutic ranges for both assays and doing counting statistics. That's always the best thing to do.
The second comment is the practical point of use. Dr. Bertina showed bad correlation in the beginning. Of course, you get bad correlation, but in practice what do you do? You give a dose of coumarin, you wait for 3 days and you do a test. If you are going to estimate on the first day, you cannot expect good correlation, but what you want to measure is the patient that is anticoagulated for several days and in that group you get the same therapeutic ranges. So, if you want to know whether you can use the chromogenic assay in practice the only thing you can do is a trial.

M. Samama : We can confirm that we have measured factor X in a large group of patients receiving coumarin derivatives and compared the results with those obtained with the thromboplastin time. We had no correlation in the beginning of our analysis. Then when we divided our patients into two groups, the short term treated patients and the long term treated patients, we found in the short term treatment no correlation and in the other group of patients the correlation was good. So, I think that if we decide to use the chromogenic method, at the beginning of the treatment we would have to perform the prothrombin time or Owren's test to determine the optimal dose of coumarin.

D. Collen : Which of course would complicate the monitoring if you have to switch from one system to another.

H.C. Hemker : I would like to comment on the remark that when you compare factor X estimations with prothrombin time estimations, you are comparing unlike things. In principle of course this is true. But already a long time ago we have shown that in a stabilized patient what is determining the prothrombin time in fact is the factor X level because that is the rate limiting factor. So, in stabilized patients you would have a better correlation than you would expect on first sight.

G. Baele : As you will see in some instances we also compared factor X determinations with S-2222 with thrombotest percentages and we have found an overall accuracy of 71 percent.

E.M. Van Wijk : I would like to ask a question to Dr. Bertina. There is a difference between the chromogenic activity of stable anticoagulated patients and the clotting activity. You are talking about decarboxy factor X. Do you think it is possible there are circulating partially carboxylated forms?

R.M. Bertina : I mentioned acarboxyfactor X and I think it is possible that there are different forms of acarboxyfactor X; maybe you should call it subcarboxylated factor X. Dr. Friberger said that acarboxyfactor X has no or a very low activity with respect to the RVV X enzyme. However, it is possible that partially carboxylated factor X molecules have a much higher contribution in the factor X assay system. Moreover we have to realize that when the contribution of acarboxyfactor X is low it will depend on the RVV X activity present in the cuvette during the assay, and this amount of RVV X has to be in excess.

H.C. Hemker : I would like to ask Dr. Friberger whether he indeed received decarboxyfactor X from Dr. Jackson or "headless" factor X which may not be the same thing. As far as I know Dr. Jackson does many experiments with "headless" factor X and hardly any, if any, with decarboxyfactor X. Then the practical point in this is, as Dr. Bertina said, that indeed the level obtained will be a function of the amount of RVV X present. As far as I could see from the graphs of Dr. Scully where the regression line intercepted the axis at 0.15, I think there will be an overall contribution of acarboxyfactor X, which amounts to about 15% of the total.

P. Friberger : I would like to answer that question. It was "headless" factor X which we tested, but maybe you can do something about this by testing acarboxyfactor X. It would be very nice to have it done and I also think that it should be checked out with the partially decarboxylated factor X and if anybody has got these preparations it would be of benefit to have it done. Then I would like to ask a question to the audience : would it be of interest in the initial phase of treatment, to determine factor VII specifically, to see what is happening with factor VII correlated to the other assays?

D. Collen : I think the answer has to be positive, hasn't it?

E.M. Van Wijk : I think the same goes for the clotting assay, because we have seen patients with 2 or 3% factor VII while the thrombotest was 6%, which is within the therapeutic range for thrombotest.

D. Collen : The question is whether a specific factor VII assay would have advantages over a specific factor X assay, especially in the initial phase of anticoagulant therapy?

P. Friberger : Maybe a research trial could answer the question whether this determination would be of benefit for routine use.

D. Collen : Do you have such a substrate?

P. Friberger : No, not at present. But it would be possible to use an assay with purified tissue factor and factor X in excess determining factor Xa activity.

L.H. Kahlé : About the measurement of factor VII, the big question is where thrombosis starts. It is known that in factor VII deficiency you can develop thrombosis. So, is it really necessary to know factor VII activity at the start or during therapy? The question we want to answer is, can you dose a patient on the basis of the factor X level, and another question, do you want to know the factor VII level because there's a risk for bleeding?

H.C. Hemker : If I have to sum up this discussion I would say that it indeed would be very interesting to have a good factor VII assay and a good factor X assay as well, and to redefine the therapeutic levels of oral anticoagulation in terms of factor VII and factor X and maybe factor II concentration. Because we should not forget that the definition of these levels in terms of prothrombin time works well in practice but still is only used because there is nothing better available; only if we can redefine these levels could we probably answer the question what factor(s) should be monitored.

D. Collen : The purpose of this meeting is to make recommendations for routine use. I think that at present assays using chromogenic substrates cannot be recommended for routine control of anticoagulant therapy.

SPECTROPHOTOMETRIC DETERMINATION OF FACTOR X WITH S-2222 IN ANTICOAGULATED AND CIRRHOTIC PATIENTS

G. BAELE

Department of Medicine, Coagulation Laboratory, University of Ghent, Ghent, Belgium.

To have an idea about the usefulness of FX determinations, with S-2222 as a chromogenic substrate, in the control of patients on oral anticoagulants, we have performed a small pilot study in 24 patients who were chronically receiving warfarin and maintained on a Thrombotest value between 6 and 15%. In a second part of our study we have looked at FX levels in cirrhotic patients.

METHODS

FX was assayed with S-2222 as outlined in the instruction leaflet of the manufacturer except that 0.2 mg/ml Russell's viper venom was used instead of 0.12 mg/ml. The end-point method was used (1). Thrombotest (Nyegaard AG, Oslo) was performed according to the manufacturer. FX was also assayed with a clotting method according to Bachmann et al. (2).

RESULTS

The levels of FX (S-2222), obtained in 24 chronically anticoagulated patients, were distressingly high (Mean : 35.2%, S.D. : 8.6%) compared to the FX:C clotting activities (Mean : 10.2%, S.D. : 4.3%) or the Thrombotest values (Mean : 10.0%, S.D. : 2.9%). However, there was no overlapping with the normal values for FX (S-2222) obtained in 30 control subjects (Mean : 99.5%, S.D. : 21.2%).

The correlation between % FX (S-2222) and % Thrombotest was statistically highly significant ($r = 0.555$, $p < 0.001$) (Fig. 1). From this relationship the percentages of FX (S-2222) were derived corresponding with 6 and 15% Thrombotest. A well controlled anticoagulant therapy level should be within the limits of 29 and 44% FX measured by the chromogenic method.

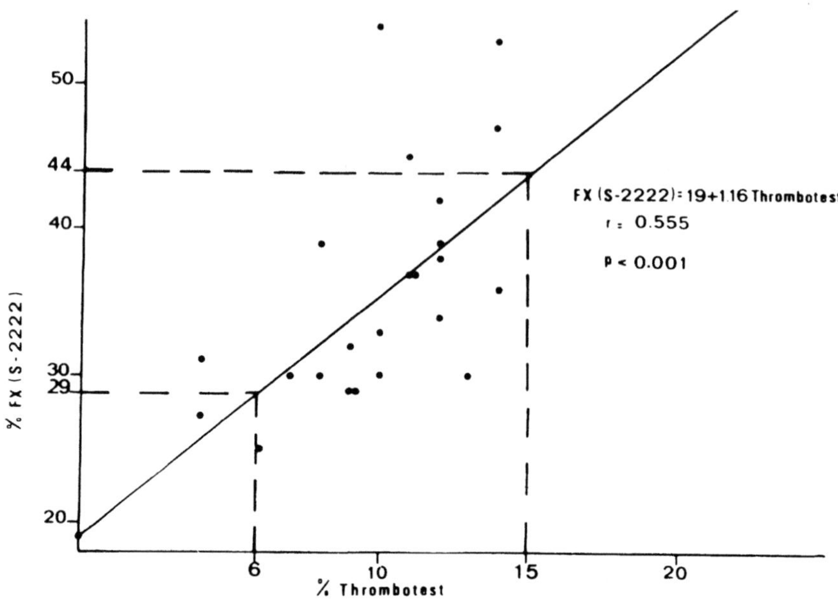

FIG. 1. Relationship between % FX (S-2222) and % Thrombotest in 24 chronically anticoagulated patients.

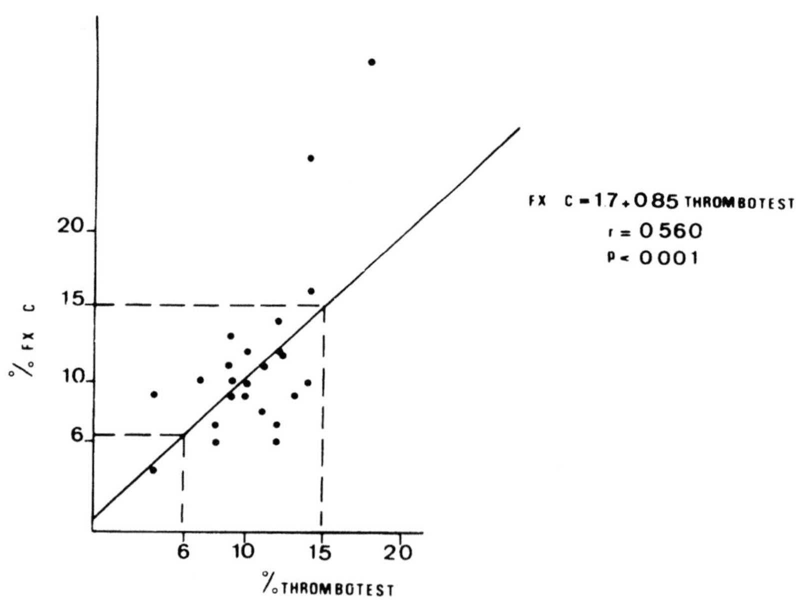

FIG. 2. Relationship between % FX:C and % Thrombotest in 24 chronically anticoagulated patients.

In an identical way FX:C percentages of 6 and 15 corresponding to Thrombotest values of 6 and 15% were obtained (Fig. 2).

The overall accuracy of the FX (S-2222) measurements compared with the Thrombotest method was 71%. The clotting assay of FX compared with the Thrombotest method scored even better : 84% (Fig. 3).

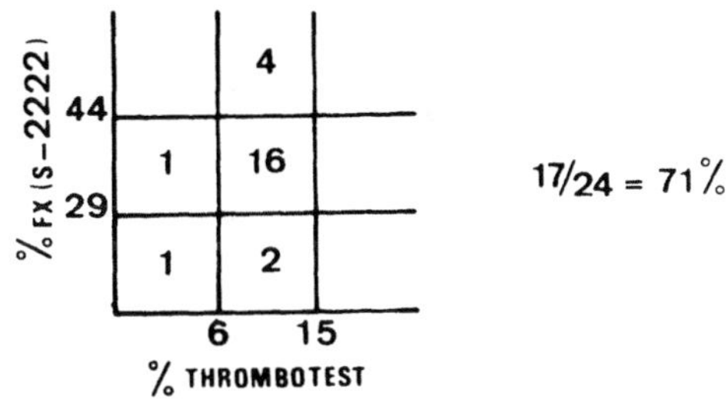

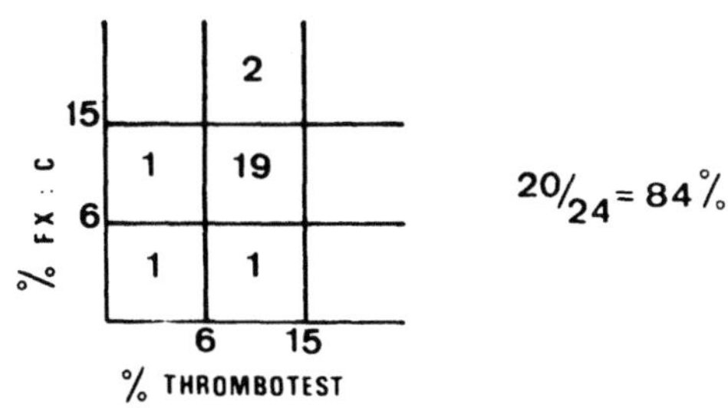

FIG. 3. Overall accuracy of the FX (S-2222) method and of the FX:C clotting assay compared with the Thrombotest method. As therapeutic ranges were considered : 6-15% with the Thrombotest method, 29-44% with the FX (S-2222) method and 6-15% with the FX:C clotting assay.

In the second part of our study FX (S-2222) levels and FX:C clotting activities were measured in 34 patients with hepatic cirrhosis. The percentages FX (S-2222) were significantly lower in the cirrhotic group than in the control group (Fig. 4). However, FX:C showed much more decreased FX levels compared to those obtained with the chromogenic substrate (Fig. 5). The correlation between % FX (S-2222) and % FX:C was highly significant ($r = 0.716$, $p < 0.001$).

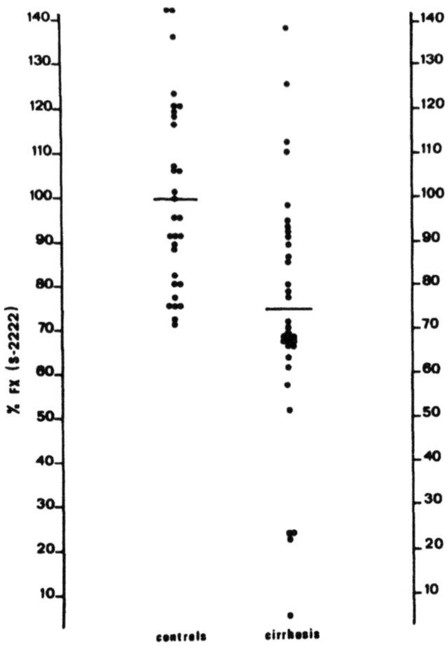

FIG. 4. FX (S-2222) in liver cirrhosis compared to control values.

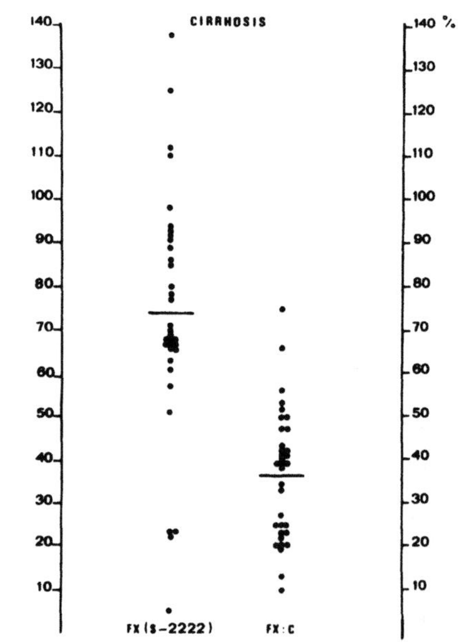

FIG. 5. Percentages FX with the chromogenic substrate S-2222 and with the clotting assay in cirrhotic patients.

DISCUSSION

The FX determination with the chromogenic substrate S-2222 has been claimed to be well suited for the monitoring of oral anticoagulants (3,4). Recently Lämmle et al. (5) reported an overall accuracy of 68% with this method if the comparison was made with a prothrombin time and a therapeutic range of 15-25% was attempted with this last technique. In the small pilot study reported here an overall accuracy of 71% comparing it with the Thrombotest method was found. The FX clotting assay scored even better. It should also be pointed out that at the beginning of coumarin therapy it is necessary to measure F VII levels to detect the initial rapid fall of F VII in order to avoid a too high coumarin dose. If one takes into account the rather low overall accuracy, the need of also measuring F VII levels at the beginning of the anticoagulant therapy and the high price of the substrate, the measurement of FX with S-2222 is presently not to be recommended in the control of patients on oral anticoagulants.

In the second part of this study FX levels were measured with the chromogenic substrate (S-2222) in 34 patients with hepatic cirrhosis. Although the FX (S-2222) levels were significantly lowered in the cirrhotic group, FX:C measured with the clotting method showed even more decreased values. An advantage of the FX determination with S-2222 is the possibility of automatisation but again the high price of the substrate is a limiting factor. As routinely performed FX determinations cannot be advocated in patients with liver cirrhosis, the role of FX assays with S-2222 seems rather limited.

SUMMARY

FX was determined with the chromogenic substrate S-2222 in a group of 24 patients who were chronically receiving warfarin. An overall accuracy of 71% was found if the comparison was made with a Thrombotest between 6 and 15%. FX (S-2222) was also measured in a group of 34 patients with hepatic cirrhosis and compared with the FX levels obtained with a FX clotting assay. The clinical need for a FX measurement with a chromogenic substrate seems rather limited.

REFERENCES

1. Aurell L, Friberger P, Karlsson G, and Claeson G. 1977. A new sensitive and highly specific chromogenic peptide substrate for factor X_a. Thromb.Res. 11, 595-609.
2. Bachmann F, Duckert F, and Koller F. 1958. The Stuart-Prower factor assay and its clinical significance. Thromb.Diathes.haemorrh. 2, 24-38.
3. Egberg N and Bergström K. 1978. Studies on assays for plasma prekallikrein and for the monitoring of coumarol therapy. Haemost. 7, 85-91.
4. Egberg N and Bergström K. 1979. Synthetic chromogenic substrates in the assay for plasma prekallikrein and coagulation factors II and X. In : Chromogenic Peptide Substrates, Chemistry and Clinical Usage. Scully MF and Kakkar VV, eds., Churchill Livingstone, Edinburgh, London and New York, pp 61-68.
5. Lämmle B, Eichlisberger R, Hänni L, Bounameaux H, Marbet GA, und Duckert F. 1979. Kontrolle der oralen Antikoagulation : Vergleich zwischen Quick- und kolorimetrischer Faktor-X-Bestimmung bei 107 Patienten. Schweiz.Med.Wschr. 109, 1115-1119.

DISCUSSION

L.H. Kahlé : I noticed that you used the RVV supplied by Wellcome in your assay. Your factor X levels are rather high, higher than other reports in the literature; in Amsterdam we only use the purified factor X activating enzyme from RVV and I think you're measuring something different from what we did?

G. Baele : Indeed, we used the RVV from Wellcome; it was not further purified.

D. Collen : Still the correlation between the results of the factor X assay and prothrombin prolongation is about the same.

G. Baele : There was no overlap with the control values in the patients on oral anticoagulants, but I agree that the levels measured were rather high.

R.M. Bertina : What type of factor X clotting assay did you use?

G. Baele : The method of Bachmann et al. which was published in 1958. They used RVV, cephalin and plasma depleted of factor VII and X by a filtrate method.

R.M. Bertina : I thought other investigators generally observed that the chromogenic factor X assay correlates well with a RVV induced clotting assay. So, indeed I am surprised that your factor X levels are much higher than you find with the clotting assay, and I think there possibly is something wrong with your chromogenic factor X assay.

G. Baele : Was that correlation also found in patients on anticoagulant therapy or only in normals?

R.M. Bertina : Yes I think so, also in patients on oral anticoagulants.

AN AUTOMATED CHROMOGENIC ANTITHROMBIN III METHOD : CLINICAL EXPERIENCE

J.W. TEN CATE

Department of Haematology, Wilhelmina Gasthuis, Amsterdam, The Netherlands.

DESCRIPTION OF THE AUTOMATED AT III ASSAY

Since 1978 an automated chromogenic method for antithrombin III (AT III) has been applied in various clinical situations in our laboratory (1).

The assay system relies on the principle that AT III in the presence of heparin inactivates thrombin, added in excess, in seconds. The remaining thrombin cleaves paranitroaniline from the chromogenic substrate S-2238. The reaction rate is calculated and the increase in absorbance per minute multiplied by a constant is then printed. The whole procedure is performed on an automated kinetic enzyme analyser.

The present assay procedure is : to 0.05 ml plasma 0.35 ml buffered saline is added. 0.005 ml diluted plasma is then incubated at 25°C for 6.0 minutes with 0.5 ml reaction buffer (0.015 M Tris, 0.015 M imidazole, 0.265 M NaCl, 0.010 M EDTA, 0.3 U/ml thrombin and 1.0 U/ml heparin). Subsequently 0.05 ml substrate S-2238 (0.8 mM) is added to the reaction mixture followed by analysis of the Δ OD/min at 405 nm.

Normal values obtained with this method in 110 EDTA plasma samples of 110 healthy volunteers were within the range of 80-140%. Reference plasma was obtained from 40 donors (sex ratio 1:1).

This method is simple, rapid and provides the thrombin inactivating activity of AT III which is the main physiological inhibitor of blood coagulation (2).

The physiological importance of AT III has initially been recognized by clinical observations in patients with congenital deficiency or defect of the AT III molecule (3,4). A decreased plasma AT III results in these conditions in recurrent thromboembolic complications. Congenital AT III deficiency is a rare phenomenon. However, acquired

AT III deficiency is a much more frequent phenomenon. Acquired deficiency states have been described to occur in 1) liver cirrhosis, 2) the nephrotic syndrome, 3) heparin therapy and 4) in disseminated intravascular coagulation (DIC).

AT III IN A GENERAL HOSPITAL PATIENT POPULATION

In order to establish the incidence of AT III deficiency, which will generally be of acquired origin, in a general hospital, we investigated 634 patients of the "Sint Lucas Hospital" in a two week period. Plasma samples were prepared from EDTA anticoagulated blood specimen, which were referred for haemoglobin estimation. Of 477 in-patients decreased AT III levels (< 80% of normal) were demonstrated to occur in 112 patients (23.5%). Of these 73 were surgical patients (65.2%). Of 157 out-patients AT III deficiency was demonstrated in 36 patients (22.9%)

AT III IN SURGICAL INTENSIVE CARE PATIENTS

Because of the unexpected high incidence of decreased AT III levels especially in surgical patients, we performed a second study in patients admitted to the surgical intensive care of our hospital. In a prospective study AT III was estimated daily in 44 consecutive patients. Of these, 11 patients revealed an uncomplicated postoperative course. 10 patients revealed complications such as cardiovascular insufficiency, bleeding episodes or pulmonary embolism. 23 patients had postoperative bacterial complications such as bronchopneumonia, wound infection, ischaemic enteritis and intra-abdominal infection. The 23 patients with bacterial infection showed a strikingly different postoperative course of AT III. The mean preoperative AT III level was 15% lower ($p < 0.05$; Wilcoxon test) and no recovery of the normal postoperative dip could be demonstrated, resulting in significantly lower AT III levels in the further postoperative course ($p < 0.05$). Summarizing these results we observed a postoperative dip between the 2nd and 5th day in all patients; in the case of postoperative bacterial complications the plasma AT III level remained low for the further period of investigation, which was ten days (5). Circulating endotoxins of gram-negative bacterial origin may be one of the main causes of acquired AT III deficiency in these patients. This may then be due to an impaired synthetic rate and/or due to increased turnover. Support for an increased AT III turnover induced by endotoxins has been revealed by animal experiments (6). Whatever the mechanism, we experienced that regular AT III estimation in this patient category may add valuable clinical information.

OBSERVATIONS IN OBSTETRICS AND IN SUBJECTS ON ORAL CONTRACEPTIVE DRUGS

The automated method for AT III is further employed on a large scale in the Department of Obstetrics in order to investigate the behaviour of AT III in obstetric patients with complications such as toxaemia, preeclampsia and with DIC. One of the interesting findings during this study was the observation of decreased AT III levels in preeclampsia (7). One of these patients admitted for preeclampsia revealed an isolated AT III deficiency of 23% as the only coagulation abnormality. The platelet count was normal. Subsequently she developed overt signs of DIC with a positive ethanol gelation test and decreasing platelets and fibrinogen. Transfusion of human AT III concentrate corrected all the abnormalities within 1 hour. She underwent uncomplicated caesarean section. This observation provides some evidence that AT III plays an important pathophysiological role in preeclampsia.

Investigation of 1000 female donors of whom about 500 were on oral contraceptive drugs revealed no deficiency of AT III. Routine investigation of AT III in subjects using the pill with low oestrogen content is therefore not advisable.

A concurrent study was performed in subjects who were treated with the "morning after" pill, which contains a high amount of oestrogen. This resulted in a decrease of AT III even up to 30% in some individuals. True AT III deficiency, i.e. values of about 50% may be observed. This should be taken into account when women are subjected to this treatment, especially with a history of thrombosis prior to treatment (8).

LIVER CIRRHOSIS

Liver cirrhosis is associated with a complex coagulation disorder which may in part be ascribed to a decreased synthesis of coagulation factors and in part to an increased turnover. Increased turnover of fibrinogen could be corrected by the intravenous administration of heparin (9). Increased turnover of prothrombin and plasminogen have also been described to occur in this condition (10). This increased turnover has been ascribed to low grade DIC. We postulated that the decreased AT III levels could be in part responsible for the observed low grade DIC. Therefore we undertook a study to evaluate the effect of human AT III concentrate transfusion upon the turnover of ^{125}I-fibrinogen (11). Complete correction of the ^{125}I-fibrinogen half-life was obtained in all seven patients who received AT III concentrate for 48 hours in the course of the turnover study. This was associated with a transient increase of plasma fibrinogen levels and of the platelet count in several patients. This study therefore provides evidence that the AT III deficiency state contributes to the occurrence of low grade DIC in liver cirrhosis.

Currently a study is performed in order to investigate the preventive effect of AT III concentrate in patients with liver cirrhosis who undergo a LeVeen shunt operation. It is well known that this procedure is complicated by DIC in the postoperative period. It has been suggested that the severity of the DIC is related to the preoperative AT III level (12).

THE NEPHROTIC SYNDROME

Acquired AT III deficiency in patients with the nephrotic syndrome has been described as the cause for the occurrence of venous thrombosis in this condition (13,14). The deficiency is due to excessive urinary excretion of AT III. It has been advised to treat these patients prophylactically with oral anticoagulants in the case of AT III deficiency which may be expected when proteinuria is about 65 mg/kg body weight/day (15). Such a close correlation between proteinuria and urinary loss of AT III was however not observed by other authors (16). We also observed two patients with AT III deficiency and nephrotic syndrome with thrombosis of respectively the renal and axillary vein. It is also our attitude to treat these patients with oral anticoagulant drugs in order to prevent thromboembolic complications.

AT III AND HEPARIN THERAPY

Prolonged intravenous administration of heparin has been reported to decrease the plasma AT III levels (17). This has recently been confirmed by others (18). Subcutaneously injected heparin did not exert such an effect as demonstrated by the same authors.

Whether this may result in recurrence of thromboembolic episodes in the course of heparin therapy has still to be revealed.

REFERENCES

1. Kahlé LH, Schipper HG, Jenkins CSP, and Ten Cate JW. 1979. An automated method for the determination of antithrombin III activity. Thromb.Res. 2, 1003-1014.
2. Abildgaard U. 1979. Evidence that antithrombin III is the main physiological inhibitor of coagulation enzymes. In : The physiological inhibitors of blood coagulation and fibrinolysis, Collen D, Wiman B, and Verstraete M (Eds.), Elsevier/North-Holland, Biomedical Press, pp 31-33.
3. Egeberg O. 1965. Inherited antithrombin deficiency causing thrombophilia. Thromb.Diath.Haemorrh. 13, 516-530.
4. Sas G, Blaskó G, Bánhegyi D, Jákó J, and Pálos LA. 1974. Abnormal antithrombin III (Antithrombin III "Budapest") as a cause of familial thrombophilia. Thromb.Diath.Haemorrh. 32, 105-115.
5. Schipper HG, Roos J, V.d. Meulen F, and Ten Cate JW. 1980. Antithrombin III deficiency in surgical intensive care patients. Submitted for publication.
6. Tanaka H, Kobayashi N, Takeuchi T, Takada M, and Malkawa T. 1979. Effect of endotoxin on kinetics of antithrombin III. Thromb.Haemostas. 42, 374.
7. Büller HR, Weenink AH, Treffers PE, Kahlé LH, Otten HA, and Ten Cate JW. 1980. Severe antithrombin III deficiency in a patient with pre-ecclampsia. Scand.J.Haemat. In Press.
8. Weenink HG, Treffers PE, and Ten Cate JW. 1980. AT III and oral contraceptive therapy. Submitted for publication.
9. Tytgat GN, Collen D, and Verstraete M. 1971. Metabolism of fibrinogen in cirrhosis of the liver. J.Clin.Invest. 50, 1690-1701.
10. Collen D, Rouvier J, Chamone DAF, and Verstraete M. 1978. Turnover of radiolabeled plasminogen and prothrombin in cirrhosis of the liver. Eur.J.Clin.Invest. 8, 185-195.
11. Schipper HG and Ten Cate JW. 1980. Antithrombin III transfusion in patients with liver cirrhosis. In : Thesis, University of Amsterdam, Schipper HG : Antithrombin III and human antithrombin III concentrates, pp 65-85.
12. Giles AR, Sauder D, Seaton TL, Johnston M, and Hirsh J. 1977. Changes in the coagulation status of patients undergoing autotransfusion of concentrated ascitic fluid as treatment of refractory ascites. Blood 50, 267.
13. Kauffmann RH, De Graeff J, and Brutel de la Rivière G. 1976. Unilateral thrombosis and nephrotic syndrome. Am.J.Med. 60, 1048-1054.

14. Kauffmann RH, Veltkamp JJ, Van Tilburg NH, and Van Es LA. 1978. Acquired antithrombin III deficiency and thrombosis in the nephrotic syndrome. Am.J.Med. 65, 607-613.
15. Thaler E, Balzar E, Kopsa H, and Pinggera WF. 1978. Acquired antithrombin III deficiency in patients with glomular proteinuria. Haemostasis 7, 257-272.
16. Jørgensen KA and Stoffersen E. 1979. Antithrombin III and the nephrotic syndrome. Scand.J.Haematol. 22, 442-448.
17. Marciniak E and Gockerman JP. 1977. Heparin-induced decrease in circulating antithrombin III. Lancet 2, 581-584.
18. Kakkar VV, Bentley PG, Scully MF, MacGregor IR, Jones NAG, and Webb PJ. 1980. Antithrombin III and heparin. Lancet 1, 103-104.

ANTITHROMBIN III AND FACTOR Xa DETERMINATION IN PATIENTS WITH LOW DOSE HEPARIN AND HIP SURGERY

T.H. SCHÖNDORF and H.G. LASCH

Zentrum für Innere Medizin am Klinikum der Justus-Liebig-Universität, 6300 Giessen, Germany.

Antithrombin III (AT III) acts as a natural coagulation inhibitor. Deficiency of AT III is associated with a tendency to deep vein thrombosis (1–3). A low concentration of AT III requires a relatively high concentration of heparin to obtain an adequate anticoagulant effect. Due to minor prophylactic effects of low dose heparin (4–7), the AT III levels and heparin activity were determined to obtain further information on the thrombophilic state in patients undergoing total hip replacement. AT III levels were assayed by two different methods and heparin activity indirectly by the factor Xa inhibitor test as an agreement has still not been reached regarding the status of AT III concentration postoperatively (8–14).

PATIENTS AND METHODS

12 female and 8 male patients with a mean age of 61 ± 9 years (range 45–72) who had been operated upon for elective hip replacement were investigated. The patients were part of a randomized trial to examine the antithrombotic effect of pre-operatively administered low-dose heparin or in combination with dextran 40 infusions.

12 additional patients (7 females and 5 males) from this trial who had developed deep vein thrombosis (DVT) diagnosed by the I-125-fibrinogen test and verified by venography or at autopsy, were evaluated. 5 of these 12 patients with DVT were infused dextran 40 in addition to the heparin prophylaxis.

METHODS

Blood samples were collected from the patients 8 hours after the last heparin injection (5,000 units s.c.), before operation and on day

1, 3 and 7./9. after the operation. The blood was diluted with 0.1 mol/l trisodium-citrate, immediately cooled and then centrifuged at 4° for 20 min at 3,000 x g.

AT III activity was determined using the thrombin susceptible substrate S-2238.

The determinations were performed according to the instructions of the manufacturer (Kabi R). A standard curve of 25% to 125% AT III activity was made for each set.

Antithrombin III (AT III, IU/ml plasma) was determined using the chromogenic substrate Tos-Gly-Pro-Arg-p-nitroaniline (Chromozym R TH, Boehringer, Mannheim). The AT III activity was controlled for each new set by Plasma-Control Plus R.

Antithrombin III protein (mg/dl) was determined by radial immunodiffusion (RID) based on the Mancini technique. Partigen R (Behringwerke, Marburg) agar gel plates containing monospecific antiserum were used. The concentrations were evaluated after 48 hours diffusion.

Statistical methods : The mean values were compared by the "t-test" (Student) for paired and unpaired samples respectively. The evaluation of correlation was based on the formula by Pearson.

RESULTS

A significant ($p < 0.05$) decrease of AT III was found on the 1st and 3rd day after the operation (Fig. 1). The reduction can be interpreted by an activation of the coagulation system as a result of extensive tissue trauma during which AT III was increasingly consumed for neutralization of enhanced amounts of activated factor X and generated thrombin.

The hypercoagulable state after hip operations - represented by reduced AT III contents - could be demonstrated by the two amidolytic assays as well as by the immunodiffusion (Fig. 1). The AT III depression persisted longer than the AT III half life of 2.8 days (15) and returned to preoperative levels on the 7th/9th day after the operation. The pronounced activation of the coagulation system is further shown by an accelerated fibrinogen-fibrin conversion rate, indicated by a tendency to shortened thrombin times after the operation (Fig. 2). In addition, the heparin levels (Table 1, Fig. 2) - determined indirectly by factor Xa-inhibition - decreased postoperatively (p not

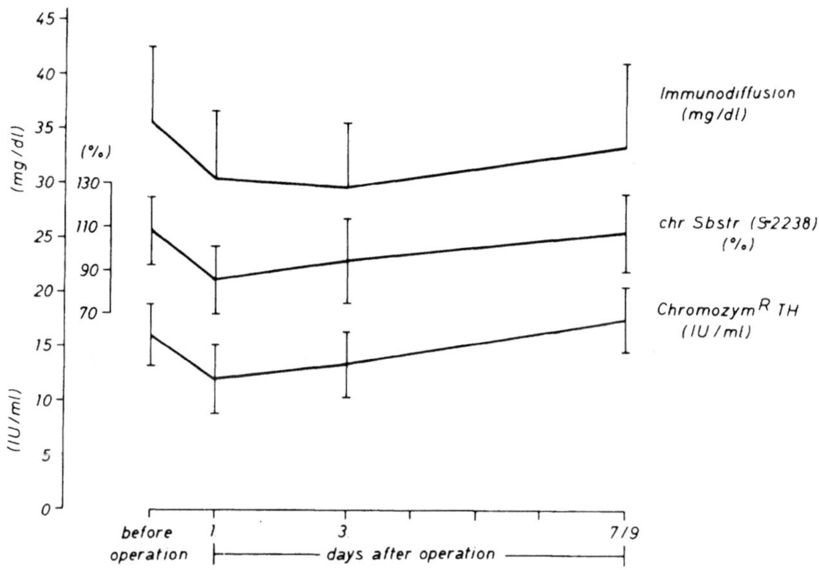

FIG. 1. Pre- and postoperative AT III determination in elective hip surgery. Significant AT III-decrease on the 1st and 3rd day after the operation.

TABLE 1.

Mean ($\bar{x}$), ± 1 standard deviation (SD) and coefficient of variation (var.) of F Xa inactivation ("heparin concentration") and PTT before and on the 1st day after elective hip surgery.

	Factor Xa (S-2222) (IU heparin/ml)		PTT (sec)	
	before operation	after operation	before operation	after operation
n	20		20	
$\bar{x}$	0.131	0.117	38.1	43.0
± 1 SD	0.069	0.072	5.7	8.7
Var.	52	61	15	20
	p = n.s.		p< 0.01	

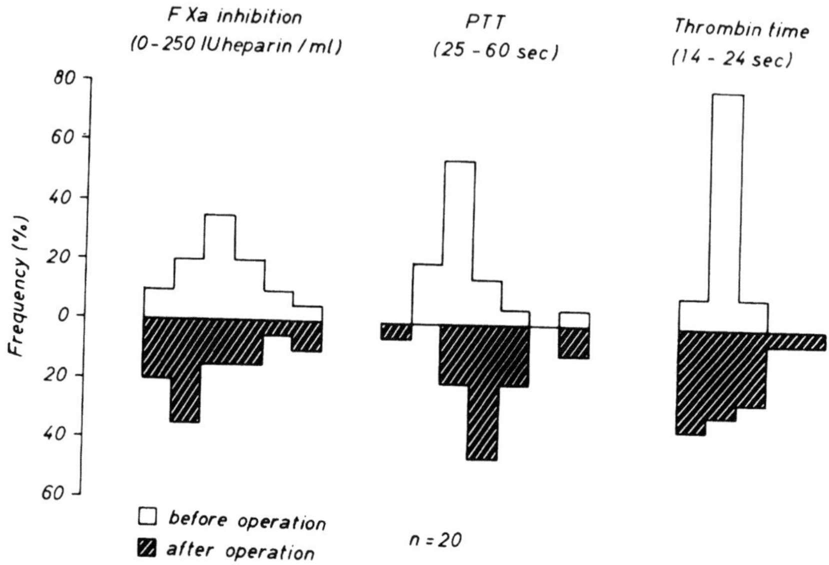

FIG. 2. Histograms of "heparin concentration" (F Xa inactivation), partial thromboplastin time (PTT) and thrombin time before and on the 1st day after the elective hip surgery.

significant). The partial thromboplastin time (PTT) was significantly prolonged only on the 1st day after the operation, but was with + 1 standard deviation still within the normal range (Table 1). The PTT prolongation could be caused by the low grade DIC with a decrease of coagulation factors. The heparin determinations (factor Xa-inhibitor test) revealed with low dose heparin prophylaxis pre- and postoperatively a wide coefficient of variation, however prolonged PTT values and higher heparin levels correlated significantly.

A significant correlation (r = 0.543) was found between the AT III activity (S- 2238) and the AT III protein before the operation (Fig. 3). Despite the parrallell, significant decrease of the AT III mean values, no correlation could be demonstrated between the two methods on the 1st day after the operation. The phenomenon of a poor correlation between two different AT III determinations was also described by other investigators in inherited AT III deficiencies (1); it could

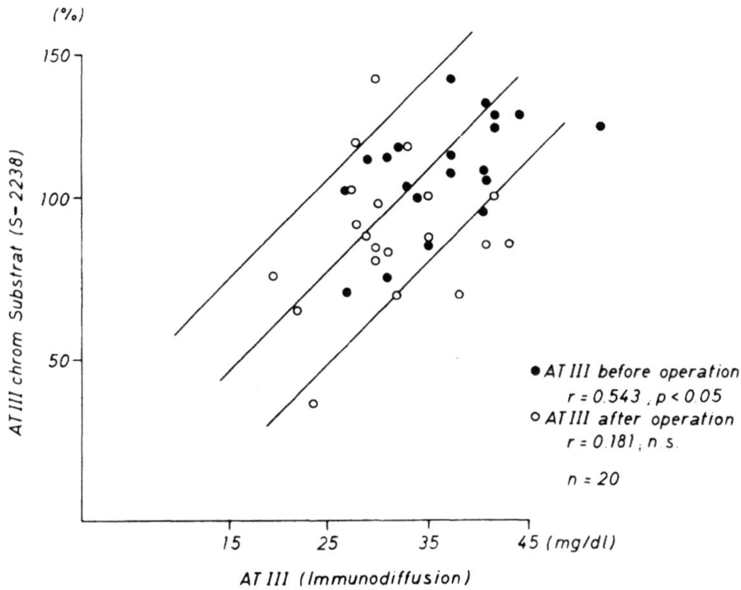

FIG. 3. Correlation between AT III determined by a chromogenic substrate (S-2238) and by immunodiffusion before and on the 1st day after hip operation.

be explained by qualitative alterations of functional sites at the AT III molecule to form various complexes with other coagulation factors (16).

Low levels of AT III ($\bar{x}$ 109 ± 13.6%; $\bar{x}$ 35.5 ± 6.1/dl) before the operation indicating a high risk of developing postoperatively DVT were not found in any of the 12 patients of the trial with subsequent DVT (Fig. 4). The distribution of lower AT III values in the histogram (Fig. 4) after the operation was more frequently found by the amidolytic method than by immunodiffusion. On the 1st or 3rd postoperative day in 7 out of the 12 patients (58%) with DVT, the AT III determined by amidolysis was lower than the 2 standard deviation range of the preoperative mean value, whereas only 2 of the 12 patients (16.6%) had an AT III protein concentration below 2 standard deviations of the mean.

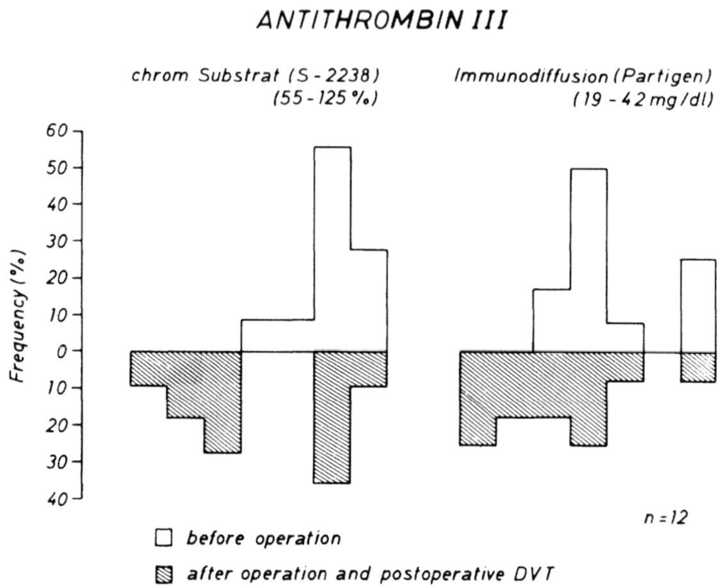

FIG. 4. Histograms of AT III determinations before and on the 1st or 3rd day after hip surgery in patients with acute postoperative deep vein thrombosis.

CONCLUSION

The significant AT III decrease demonstrated in the present study by two different methods can be considered as a contributing factor for the high susceptibility to develop DVT after hip replacement operations. The determination of the AT III activity by an amidolytic assay can be rapidly performed and was more frequently associated with postoperative thrombosis than significantly reduced AT III contents determined by radial immunodiffusion. However, the finding of low functional AT III content is only an additional indicator of an underlying DVT and was absent in more than 40% of the patients despite acute DVT.

The low AT III levels and decreased "heparin" concentrations (FXa) support the thesis by Wessler (17) "for a greater heparin dose requirement after hip reconstructions" to improve the prophylactic effect.

REFERENCES

1. Sas G, Blasko G, Banhegyi D, Jako J, and Palos LA. 1976. Abnormal antithrombin III (Antithrombin III "Budapest") as a cause of familial thrombophilia. Thrombos.Diathes.haemorrh. 32, 105-115.
2. Lechner K, Thaler E, Niessner H, Nowotny C, and Partsch H. 1977. Antithrombin-III-Mangel und Thromboseneigung. Wiener Klin.Wschr. 89, 215-222.
3. Lane JL and Biggs R. 1977. The natural inhibitors of coagulation: antitrombin III, heparin cofactor and antifactor Xa. In : Recent Advances in Blood Coagulation - 2, Poller L (Ed), Churchill Livingstone, Edinburgh, pp 123-139.
4. Hampson WGJ, Harris FC, Keith LH, Roberts PH, McCall IW, Jackson PC, Powell NL, and Staddon GE. 1974. Failure of low-dose heparin to prevent deep-vein thrombosis after hip-replacement arthroplasty. Lancet 2, 795-797.
5. Kakkar VV. 1978. The current status of low-dose heparin in the prophylaxis of thrombophlebitis and pulmonary embolism. World J.Surg. 2, 3-18.
6. Schnyder M and Gruber UF. 1977. Prophylaxe postoperativer tiefer Venenthrombosen in der elektiven Hüftchirurgie. Akt.Traumatol. 7, 275-279.
7. Schöndorf TH. 1979. Heparin therapy in orthopedic surgery. In : Etat actuel de la prévention des accidents thromboemboliques postopératoires par l/héparinothérapie sous-cutanée à faible doses. Exerpta Medica, pp 56-63.
8. Aberg M, Nilsson IM, and Hedner U. 1973. Antithrombin III after operation. Lancet 2, 1337.
9. Donati MB, Vandenberghe K, Molla A, De Roo M, and Verstraete M. 1973. Postoperative antithrombin III. Lancet 1, 726-727.
10. Stathakis N, Papayannis AG, and Gardikas SCD. 1973. Postoperative antithrombin III concentration. Lancet 1, 430.
11. Hedner U and Nilsson IM. 1973. Antithrombin III in a clinical material. Thromb.Res. 3, 631-641.
12. Bergström K and Lahnborg G. 1975. The effect of major surgery, low doses of heparin and thromboembolism on plasma antithrombin. Comparison of immediate thrombin inhibiting capacity and the antithrombin III content. Thromb.Res. 6, 223-233.
13. Schöndorf TH and Hey D. 1975. Wirksamkeit von subkutan verabreichtem Heparin zur Thromboseprophylaxe bei grossen Hüftgelenksoperationen. Dtsch.Med.Wschr. 100, 2014-2018.
14. Sagar S, Nair D, Stamatakis JD, Maffei FH, Higgins AF, Thomas DP, and Kakkar VV. 1976. Efficacy of low-dose heparin in prevention of extensive deep-vein thrombosis in patients undergoing total-hip replacement. Lancet 1, 1151-1154.
15. Collen D, Schetz J, De Cock F, Holmer E, and Verstraete M. 1977. Metabolism of antithrombin III (heparin cofactor) in man : effects of venous thrombosis and of heparin administration. Eur.J.Clin. Invest. 7, 27-35.
16. Andersson LO, Engmean L, and Henningsson E. 1977. Crossed immunoelectrophoresis as applied to studies on complex formation. The binding of heparin to antithrombin III and the antithrombin III-thrombin complex. J.Immunol.Methods 14, 271-281.
17. Wessler S. 1975. Mini-dose heparin. Thrombos.Diathes.haemorrh. 34, 718-726.

DISCUSSION

M. Samama : We also use an automated method for antithrombin III determination; the apparatus is a Gilford 3500. A test is performed in about 7 sec. The correlation with the immunological method was very good (r = 0.76). We studied normal subjects and patients with a congenital deficiency not receiving treatment or coumarin derivatives. The mean in congenital deficiency is not very low, about 67-68%. We have found many years ago and this has been reported at the Phoenix meeting by the American haematologists, that during treatment with L-asparaginase in leukaemic patients there is a very important decrease in antithrombin III levels. The other results are in good correlation with the ones already published. The last finding was that in diabetic patients with background retinopathy we found a significant increase in antithrombin III using this method.

D. Collen : At this stage we should discuss two questions. Firstly, what are the clinical indications for measuring antithrombin III, and secondly, which of the assays available is the method of choice? Besides the chromogenic method there are of course other procedures which however seem to be more complicated.

L. Wijnja : Dr. ten Cate, in internal medicine we find low levels of AT III in liver insufficiency and in the literature also low levels of AT III are mentioned in the nephrotic syndrome. Did you find low levels of AT III in the nephrotic syndrome and if you did, in what type of nephrotic syndrome, and what was the duration of the illness?

J.W. ten Cate : We had a single case of proteinuria, associated with acquired AT III deficiency and thrombotic complications after kidney transplantation. But we did not perform a systematic study in patients with the nephrotic syndrome. There is more information in a recent study from Vienna.

T.H. Schöndorf : As you mentioned there is a study by Thaler et al. from Vienna (Haemostasis 1978, 7: 257-272). They found a pronounced AT III depression in nephrotic syndrome when the proteinuria is more than 5 gram protein per day, otherwise it is probably compensated.

J.W. ten Cate : I am of the opinion that it has to be a proteinuria of 5 grams for a prolonged period before a deficiency state develops, which may also depend upon the synthetic capacity of the liver.

T.H. Schöndorf : I think that at the beginning AT III levels might be compensated but in the study by Thaler and another by Kaufman (Amer.J.Med. 1978, 65: 607) they didn't state how long the proteinuria lasted.

H.A. Holm : It is also our experience that AT determination is helpful in the diagnosis of liver disease. In hematology it is useful for the diagnosis of DIC, and in general AT III assays are helpful in patients where you don't have a certain diagnosis. This also implies the consideration of therapy. As mentioned by Dr. ten Cate about "toxemic" women, we have the same experience in a case where the toxemia led to an AT III value of 23%, and this situation was corrected after infusion of antithrombin. Complete cure followed.

Cl. Bouvier : This is the only chromogenic assay that we use almost routinely, and exactly as Dr. ten Cate and Dr. Holm said: in sepsis, in acute hepatitis, in hemolytic uraemic syndrome it is very useful to have the AT III determination. I would even go a little further than Dr. ten Cate : the rapid recovery of AT III in DIC seems to be associated with a better prognosis.

J.W. ten Cate : Indeed, in patients with liver cirrhosis it is of great practical and clinical importance to treat complicating DIC, associated with a haemorrhagic diathesis on the basis of the AT III concentration. We were able to do some clinical studies in patients with an untreatable bleeding tendency under these circumstances. We found extremely low levels of AT III and we could help these patients after administration of either fresh frozen plasma or occasionally human AT III concentrates in combination with heparin. Other indications for the AT III estimation at present are DIC in general to understand the type of DIC, patients with thrombosis or thromboembolic complications and I'd like to suggest to screen for AT III in the course of i.v. heparin therapy.

D. Collen : I will sum up the possible indications for AT III determination which have been presented. It could be used to evaluate liver function, in haemolytic uraemic syndrome, in acute hepatitis, during heparin therapy, during bacteremia or septicemia, in nephrotic syndrome, in post-operative patients, in disseminated intravascular coagulation, in thrombosis, in critically ill patients and in toxemia. Could we now evaluate these indications critically and make a suggestion in which conditions it is strongly advisable to do AT III determinations, and in which conditions it may add some useful information but is not necessary for either diagnosis or treatment of the patient.

J.J. Sixma : Dr. ten Cate, did you ever see low AT III in a liver patient who did not have a very prolonged prothrombin time?

J.W. ten Cate : That is true. It does not add any more information about the synthetic capacity of the liver.

J.J. Sixma : The group of patients is however very large.

T.H. Schöndorf : Maybe one has to investigate the importance of low AT III for DIC and not only as a sign of reduced synthetic liver capacity. Depending upon the possibilities of your laboratory you can demonstrate DIC by demonstrating fibrin monomers. Reduced AT III levels may with other coagulation tests and decreased platelet number support the diagnosis of DIC and may be helpful to decide on a substitution therapy and/or heparin administration.

J.J. Sixma : Dr. ten Cate, have you ever seen a considerably reduced AT III level but a normal fibrinogen level in DIC, liver disease excepted?

J.W. ten Cate : I think it is too early to define exactly in which patient groups we have to know the AT III level. Maybe we should wait for another 2 or 3 years because where clinical chemists have now experience with sodium and potassium for 20 years, this is still a new and expanding area.

D. Collen : Is deep vein thrombosis in a patient an indication for an AT III determination? Only 1% of these patients will have a lowered AT III level. Is it useful to screen a hundred to find one, and will this have any therapeutic implications?

M. Samama : I would say that in young patients with unexplained phlebitis the AT III evaluation must be performed before any anticoagulant therapy.

D. Collen : Should deep vein thrombosis be considered as an indication for AT III determination?

H.A. Holm : A limited group of patients with DVT may be tested for AT III levels but not as a general rule. Although, as pointed out, antithrombin levels are regularly decreased during heparin infusion, and we have seen that in 10 percent of a group of 200 patients the AT III levels were below 70 percent. But I would say that this does not imply that one should monitor these patients on their AT III levels, because we cannot tell what the practical implications are.

D. Collen : Do you ever see patients during heparin therapy, not DIC or severe synthetic deficiencies, but regular patients on heparin therapy for pulmonary embolism or DVT with such decrease in AT III that interferes with the heparin therapy?

H.A. Holm : Maybe patients with malignancy have low AT III levels because of liver metastasis and in these cases the hypercoagulable state is almost impossible to control with heparin. In instances like that it might be useful to know the AT III level.

D. Collen : So, again in selected cases.

T.H. Schöndorf : Diseases with renal or intestinal protein loss might be important to determine AT III regularly. Secondly we have the results after gynecological operations where there were no alterations in contrast to hip operations. In general, I think one should be selective with the AT III determination. Another selective indication for an AT III determination is during treatment with AT III concentrates (Thaler E. et al., Thrombos.Haemostas. 1979, 42: 249; Schipper H.G. et al., Thrombos.Haemostas. 1979, 42: 249).

D. Collen : In order to raise a patient from 70 to 100 percent AT III, the equivalent of about 2 liters of plasma or approximately 500 mg AT III is required.

T.H. Schöndorf : This was only a prospective thought because as I demonstrated a very pronounced depression was only found in about 58% of the patients, below the 2 standard deviation, and eventually it would be necessary to replace AT III in these patients.

G. Baele : I think that in liver cirrhosis the clinical value of AT III determinations depends also on the value of AT III concentrates in treatment. Much more experience on this point is certainly needed.

Question from the audience : What should be done about toxemia patients that have very low AT III levels?

J.W. ten Cate : This is difficult to answer because there are no exact data on patients with such low AT III levels and toxemia is a dangerous situation and occasionally fatal. I think, after the recent publication of Kakkar, it could be tried to treat these patients with heparin subcutaneously because he observed no further decrease of AT III. I know that this level of AT III is associated with high risk for thromboembolic complications; such a situation plus surgery i.e. cesarian section, plus progressive DIC, plus kidney function abnormalities was for us an indication to treat the patient with AT III concentrate. How to treat I cannot answer. Maybe I would prefer subcutaneous heparin, I have no answer actually.

D. Collen : Everybody agrees that the chromogenic substrate for AT III is the method of choice above the clotting or immunologic methods.

HEPARIN CONCENTRATION (S-2222) AND EFFECT OF HEPARIN TREATMENT (BLEEDING COMPLICATIONS, PULMONARY EMBOLISM AND CLEARING OF THE THROMBUS)

H.A. HOLM, U. ABILDGAARD, F. LAERUM and T. WOLLAND
Medical Department A, Aker Hospital, Oslo, Norway.

A wide number of laboratory tests have been used to monitor heparin therapy. Until now these tests have been variations of clotting assays. Introduction of chromogenic substrates means that a new tool is at hand for monitoring heparin therapy.

The clinician has at least three important requirements for what we would call the ideal test for monitoring heparin therapy. The test should be easy to perform; the cost should be low, and above all we would like a test with high sensitivity and high specificity with respect to the ability of identifying patients in danger of bleeding, or threathened by pulmonary embolism.

Although the two first requirements are extremely important, they will not be dealt with in the following account. It is the third requirement I will focus on for the rest of this presentation.

The data presented in this report are preliminary findings from a cooperative study involving 14 Norwegian hospitals. The clinical part of the study has been terminated, and we are now working with the patient records and preparing the final statistical analysis, which we hope, will give us a more rational basis for selection of dose regimens and tests to be applied for monitoring heparin therapy.

The present data are based on material comprising 237 patients with phlebographically proven DVT treated with heparin infusion for 5-7 days. The recommended dose was 150 U/kg followed by 400 U/kg/24 hours, bearing in mind that this dose should be reduced in elderly people, and especially in elderly women. Blood samples were drawn once daily. Most of the hospitals involved in this study did not use any assay for monitoring heparin therapy prior to this study, and the results of the heparin assays were mostly not available at the time it would be of any consequence to the patient.

The following four heparin assays were performed :

a) Amidolytic assay with the chromogenic substrate S-2222, Coatest heparin (1) .

b) APTT with the Cephotest method.

c) Thrombin time with citrated plasma and buffer (2).

d) Thrombin time combined with recalcification (3).

Any sign and type of bleeding was recorded daily by the clinician in charge. The criteria for classifying a bleeding episode as major were : 1) fatal bleeding,

2) blood loss which required blood transfusion,

3) blood loss which caused functional deterioration (e.g. pareses, severe pain).

Major bleeding episodes were recorded in 7 patients, one of which was fatal (caused by a thoracocentesis). Five had retroperitoneal bleeds, and one a haematemesis. Except for traumatic bleeding, blood loss occurred late in the therapeutic period, mainly on the 4th or 5th day.

Of 20 patients with minor bleeding episodes, 10 had skin or mucosal haemorrhages, 6 macroscopic haematuria, and 4 signs of gastrointestinal bleeding.

In order to see if the major bleeding complications could be predicted by any of the heparin assays employed, we compared the percentage of blood samples with heparin values above the "therapeutic range" in patients with major blood loss, with the percentage of samples above "therapeutic range" in the total material (Table 1).

TABLE 1.

Relation major bleeding complications/heparin activities

Test	Per cent of blood samples with heparin values above "therapeutic range" (> 0.7 U/ml) Major bleeding	Total material
Amidolytic assay (S-2222)	69	16
APTT (Cephotest)	38	12
Thrombin time	22	7
Thrombin time ($CaCl_2$)	34	6
	"sensitivity"	"specificity"

The therapeutic range was defined as 0.2-0.7 U/ml, which has been the range commonly accepted for full dose heparin therapy in our country. To express the activity assay in units of heparin rather than in seconds, the clotting times were "transformed" into units of heparin using standard curves of normal pooled plasma.

As you see from Table 1, almost 70 per cent of the blood samples from patients suffering from major blood loss, had a heparin activity indicating overdosage according to the amidolytic assay. This patient group is also "identified" by the clotting assays, but to a lesser extent. On the other hand, the thrombin time methods showed a higher "specificity" than the amidolytic assay.

TABLE 2.
Relation minor bleedings/heparin concentration (S-2222)

Type of bleeding	N	Per cent of blood samples with heparin values above "therapeutic range" (> 0.7 U/ml)
Skin/mucosa	10	57
Macroscopic haematuria	6	23
Gastrointestinal	4	18
Total material	237	16

Table 2 gives the relation between minor bleedings and the heparin concentration (S-2222). The patients with skin or mucosal haemorrhage clearly had a higher heparin concentration compared to the total patient group, while patients with macroscopic haematuria or signs of gastrointestinal bleeding (without fall in haemoglobin) did not differ from the total group with respect to heparin concentration.

Pulmonary embolism was recorded in 9 patients (3.8%), of which none proved fatal. The diagnosis was based on clinical criteria, and the low incidence is well in accordance with the concept that heparin is effective in prevention of pulmonary embolism.

Table 3 gives the relation between pulmonary embolism and heparin activity with respect to subtherapeutic values, that is below 0.2 U/ml. As you see from the left column, subtherapeutic values occurred in 73 per cent of the blood tests according to amidolytic assay in

TABLE 3.

Relation pulmonary embolism/heparin activities

Test	Per cent of blood samples with heparin values below "therapeutic range" (< 0.2 U/ml) Pulmonary embolism	Total material
Amidolytic assay (S-2222)	73	28
APTT (Cephotest)	71	48
Thrombin time	22	7
Thrombin time ($CaCl_2$)	34	6
	"sensitivity"	"specificity"

patients with pulmonary embolism, compared to 28 per cent in the total material. The "sensitivity" of the Cephotest with respect to pulmonary embolism is also high, but its "specificity" (right column) is rather poor. Again, the two thrombin time methods have a rather low "sensitivity", but their "specificity" is good.

Although the role of heparin is well established with respect to prevention of pulmonary embolism, little is known about its influence on the fate of the thrombus. Table 4 compares the results of control phlebography and mean heparin concentration in a limited number of patients. Two roentgenologists have compared the first and second phlebography and divided the patients into four categories : increased thrombosis, unchanged, partly cleared and normalized. There seems to be a clear tendency towards improvement the higher the mean heparin concentration. This could imply that the patient would be better off with a higher heparin dose, as long as it does not cause bleeding complications.

TABLE 4.

Results of control phlebography and relation to heparin concentration (S-2222)

Control phlebography	N	Heparin conc. (U/ml) mean	S.D.
Increased thrombosis	22	.26	(.25)
Unchanged	38	.35	(.32)
Partly cleared	40	.47	(.36)
Normalized	2	.89	(.38)

Before arriving at my final conclusions it should be pointed out that the results presented are based on a preliminary analysis of the material. Furthermore, practical problems concerning the reliability of infusion pumps and so forth, have not been mentioned at all. From our material we have got a clear impression that the day to day variation in heparin activities in many instances exceeds that which can be explained by dose variation alone. A constant infusion is mandatory if one is to obtain the full benefit from heparin assays. In cases of uncontrolled dose variations, the answer you get, may be more misleading than guiding.

With these reservations, the conclusions which may be drawn from our preliminary analysis, are that

1) major bleeding episodes were associated with high heparin concentration and high heparin activity;
2) pulmonary embolism was associated with low heparin concentration and low heparin activity;
3) clearing of the thrombus was related to the heparin concentration;
4) amidolytic assay seems to give the best overall correlation ("sensitivity" and "specificity") with the in vivo effects of heparin.

REFERENCES

1. Teien AN and Lie M. 1977. Evaluation of an amidolytic heparin assay method : Increased sensitivity by adding purified antithrombin III. Thromb.Res. 10, 399-410.
2. Kierulf P. 1971. Heparin. Virkemåte, indikasjoner, administrasjon. T. norske Lægeforen 91, 2105-2108.
3. Denson KWE and Bonnar J. 1973. The measurement of heparin. A method based on the potentiation of anti-factor Xa. Thromb.Diath. Haemorrh. 30, 471-479.

DISCUSSION

<u>H.R. Lijnen</u> : Did you study the influence of different types, different molecular weight forms of heparin in this assay?

<u>H.A. Holm</u> : No, we did not.

<u>W.G. Van Aken</u> : Did you take into account in your analysis the localisation of the thrombus, whether it is proximal or confined to the calf?

H.A. Holm : No, we are now preparing a full statistical analysis and then the localisation of the thrombus will come into the picture.

W.G. Van Aken : Would you agree that a number of patients in which the thrombus apparently extended when you looked at the phlebography, were perhaps mainly proximal vein thrombi, and that possibly we have to take into account that for those patients the regimen might be different than for the patients with calf DVT?

H.A. Holm : Yes, that might be possible. But all the same, there is a tendency as we saw for the heparin concentration to increase with clearing of the thrombus. And when you look at the localisation of the thrombus, it is possible that people that get improvement of their legs may have had an embolus to the lung. I think, however, that these arguments do not interfere with the concept that there might be a relation between heparin concentration and clearing of the thrombus.

W.G. Van Aken : When was the second phlebography performed?

H.A. Holm : When heparin was discontinued or the day after.

W.G. Van Aken : Were these patients treated with oral anticoagulants from the beginning or at a later phase in the treatment?

H.A. Holm : Treatment with warfarin was started after 3 days of heparin, just to avoid the problem you probably thought of now.

D. Thomas : Do you really have the data to support your third conclusion? You don't have to be a statistician to see there is no statistically significant difference between the levels that you quoted; you have only 2 patients.

H.A. Holm : I agree with you that there are only 2 patients that had complete clearing of the thrombus and that is too low a number to say anything. But I think this is more than an impression, but until full statistical analysis is performed, I will not hold for sure that this is the truth.

D. Collen : Would you advise to monitor heparin therapy on a routine base?

H.A. Holm : Yes, I think it is feasible to guide dose adjustment. But the technical side of the problem has to be discussed too : you must give a continuous infusion. If not, you might get values that actually are nonsens.

D. Collen : Is there a major advantage in sensitivity, and discrimination between sub- and over-dose of heparin with the amidolytic assay as compared to APTT?

H.A. Holm : No, I would not call it major. According to our results Cephotest is useful in this respect too.

M. Samama : What in your country is the range for Cephotest that is estimated to be dangerous for haemorrhage, which is the therapeutic range?

H.A. Holm : According to the manufacturer it is 2 to 4 times the values obtained in normal plasma. Four times may be a little high.

W.G. Van Aken : Your material is mainly composed of postoperative patients, or are also medical patients included?

H.A. Holm : It is a mixture of surgical and medical patients, comprising more medical than surgical patients.

THE FIBRINOLYTIC SYSTEM

FUNCTIONAL ASSAYS OF THE COMPONENTS OF THE FIBRINOLYTIC SYSTEM USING A PLASMIN SENSITIVE SUBSTRATE - A REVIEW*.

P. FRIBERGER AND M. KNÖS

Kabi AB, Peptide Research, Mölndal, Sweden.

This is a short review and update on methods for plasmin, antiplasmin, plasminogen (PLG), and plasminogen activators and the assay conditions are presented elsewhere (1-4). Therefore we will try to concentrate on critical points in the assays. Suggestions for future work in this field will also be included.

PLASMIN STANDARDIZATION

Plasmin activity has usually been determined by using casein or fibrin as substrate. Casein is, however, by no means a natural plasmin substrate and it is a rather unselective protease substrate as well. The natural plasmin substrate, fibrin, is difficult to handle and is not so frequently used for plasmin standardization.

Probably because of the difficulties with these macromolecular substrates, small synthetic substrates like lysine and arginine esters and amides seem, hitherto, more accepted in fibrinolysis than in e.g. coagulation assays. Among these amino acid derivatives, the esters are rather unselective and the amides are quite insensitive. Substrate affinity as well as the selectivity have been increased by replacing the single amino acid by e.g. a tripeptide chain. By trial and error it was found that lysine as expected was the best C-terminal amino acid, that leucine, proline or phenylalanine in position 2 is favourable and that an unsubstituted D amino acid in position 3 increases both the sensitivity and the solubility of the substrate.

The substrate S-2251 (D-Val-Leu-Lys-pNA) is a rather sensitive substrate for plasmin. Although a potency of 10 less sensitive than the

* Some of the tables and figures are taken from earlier publications in Chromogenic Peptide Substrates and in Progress in Chemical Fibrinolysis and Thrombolysis Vol IV (see References).

TABLE 1

THE SENSITIVITY OF AVAILABLE SUBSTRATES

	Trypsin	Thrombin	Factor Xa	Plasma kallikrein	Glandular kallikrein	Plasmin	Urokinase
S-2160	0.150	0.140	0.002	0.004	0.001	0.002	0.001
S-2222	0.730	0.005	0.200	0.005	0.003	0.006	0.007
S-2238	0.270	0.480	0.008	0.007	0.004	0.002	0.002
S-2251	0.030	0.002	0.001	0.007	0.020	0.040	0.000
S-2266	0.110	0.005	0.001	0.006	0.130	0.002	0.001
S-2302	0.070	0.030	0.040	0.190	0.100	0.040	0.000
S-2444	0.620	0.003	0.004	0.001	0.001	0.001	0.040

By using 4.10^{-9} mol/l of enzyme, the activities A/min given in the table are obtained. The conditions used are those optimal for the combination for which the substrate has been designed. $\{S_o\} = 2.K_m$ except for S-2160 and S-2238 where $\{S_o\} = 0.1$ mmol/l.

best combinations of enzyme-chromogenic substrates, its sensitivity is excellent for all practical purposes. The selectivity also seems adequate even if glandular kallikrein and trypsin split the substrate at a considerable rate (on molar bases 50 and 75% that of plasmin). Coagulation factors as well as plasminogen activators do not hydrolyze S-2251 much (Table 1-3), at least not at the pH and ionic strength optimal for plasmin (5,6). The somewhat high activities of human tissue activator on the -Lys-pNA substrates (Table 3) have been explained by the existance of some minor enzymatic impurities in the preparation used.

TABLE 2
The sensitivity of available substrates

	UK	TA	PLG-SK	Pli	
S-2160	0.5	0.5	2.4	1.5	140 (Thr)
S-2238	2.0	1.7	2.9	2.2	480 (Thr)
S-2222	7.4	9.6	0.6	6.0	200 (FXa)
S-2266	0.9	1.5	19	2.3	130 (Gl.kal.)
S-2302	0.4	1.3	52	40	190 (Pl.kal.)
S-2251	0.3	1.2	59	40	
S-2444	41	6.3	6.4	1.3	
S-2322	19	12	0.3	1.0	

By using 4.10^{-9} mol/l of enzyme, the activities mA/min given in the table are obtained. The conditions used are those optimal for the combination for which the substrate has been designed $\{S_o\} = 2.K_m$ except for S-2160 where and S-2238 where $\{S_o\} = 0.1$ mmol/l.

As plasmin is a rather unstable enzyme, measures have been taken to stabilize it. Glycerol (50%) and low pH (3-4) without buffer capacity are excellent stabilizors and Carbowax^R 6000 (0.5%) protects the protein from absorption to e.g. glass surfaces.

The plasmin solution should be kept at room temperature for 1/2 h before analysis and special care must be taken when pipetting the viscous glycerol-containing solution.

The conditions for plasmin assay have been optimized (1). pH = 7.4 (Fig. 1) and ionic strength 0.15 (Fig. 2) has been recommended. These optima are not sharp. Among different buffers tested (Tris,

TABLE 3

THE SENSITIVITY OF AVAILABLE SUBSTRATES

Substrate \ Enzyme	Urokinase HMW	Urokinase LMW	Tissue activator Porcine	Tissue activator Human	Vascular activator	Plg-SK	Plasmin
H - <Glu - Gly - Arg - pNA (S-2444)	<u>100</u>	<u>100</u>	125	65	160	10	20
H-D-<Glu " " "	85	85	50	55	120	9	6
H-D- Glu - " " "	55	65	30	25	70	10	9
H-D- Val - " " " (S-2322)	35	35	<u>100</u>	<u>100</u>	<u>100</u>	15	9
H - <Glu - Ala - Arg - "	55	55	155	185	155	30	40
H-D- Ile - Pro - " "	50	50	190	235	180	35	110
H-D- Phe - Aze - " "	35	20	140	215	165	30	70
H - <Glu - Pro - " "	60	55	175	205	255	215	315
H-D- Val - Leu - Lys - " (S-2251)	15	3	20	115	100	<u>100</u>	<u>100</u>
H-D- Val - Phe - " "	8	1	20	80	130	80	110
H - <Glu - " " "	15	4	35	200	220	195	320

Each enzyme is standardized against one substrate (100). No direct comparison between the columns is possible because different amounts of the enzymes are used. $\{S_o\}$ = 0.4 mmol/l.

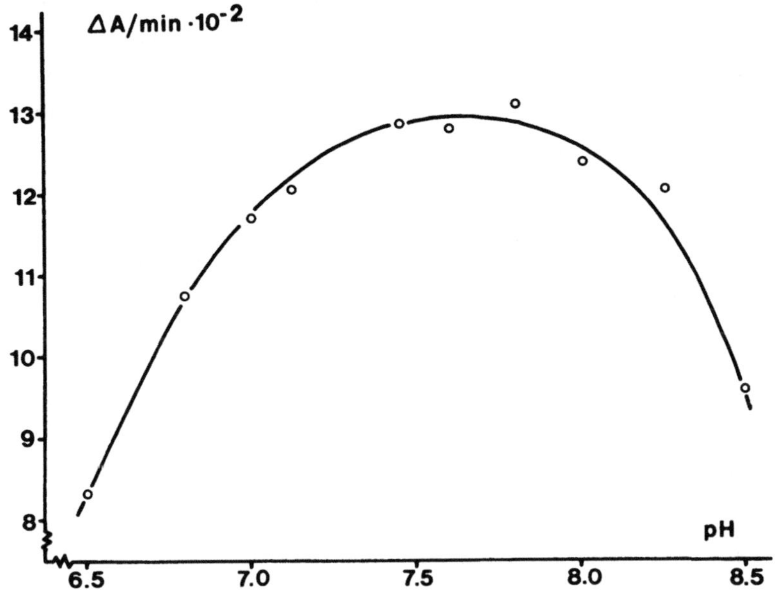

FIG. 1. Plasmin activity in Tris buffer, I=0.15 at different pH.

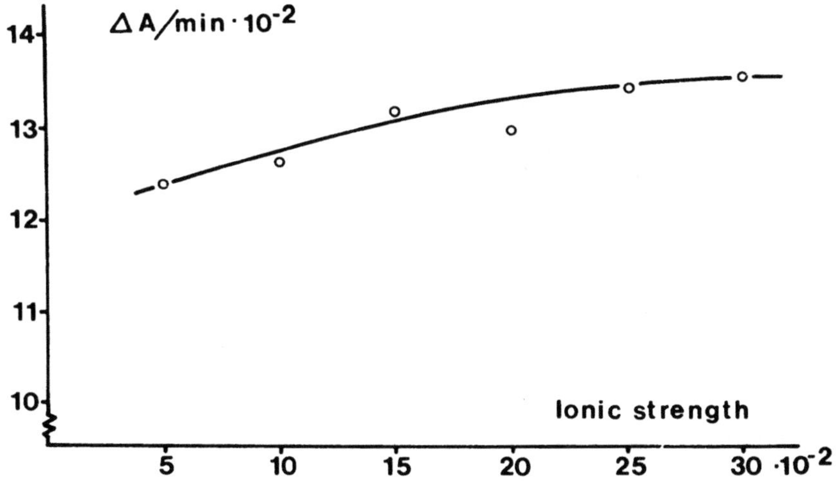

FIG. 2. Plasmin activity in Tris buffer pH 7.4 at different ionic strength (I).

Tris-Imidazol, Phosphate, Veronal and TES) Tris was preferred. The activity increases approximately linearly with the temperature (20-40°C) and with approximately 2% per °C. For human plasmin we found a K_m = 0.26 and 0.25 mmol/l and V=0.49 and 0.53 µmol/min.unit for the Kabi (CU) and British standard (U) respectively. The porcine plasmin from Novo (NU) gave a K_m=0.37 mmol/l and V=3.80 µmol/min.unit.

Additions of reasonable amounts of substances like lysine, EACA, glycerol, and DMSO interfere with plasmin by increasing its activity measured with S-2251.

In our hands repeated determinations give a C.V. of less than 2% (n = 10). Between days, equipment or laboratories, a larger variation is expected but will be reduced by using a pNA standard solution and by a careful calibration of the temperature in the cuvette.

Standard curves on three different plasmins are shown in Fig. 3.

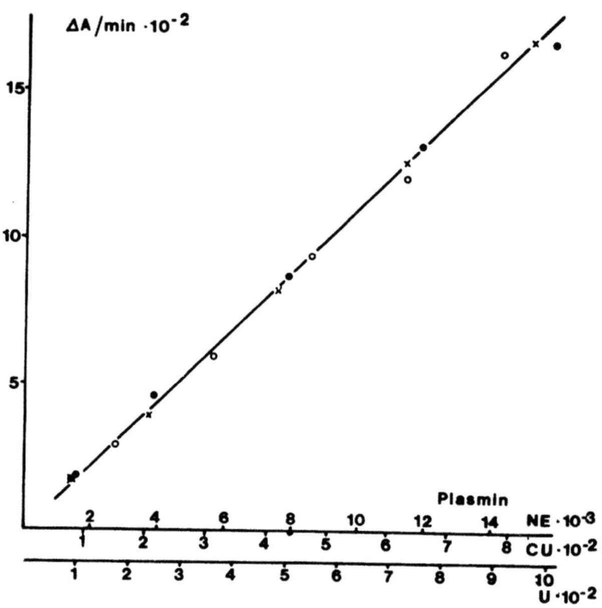

FIG. 3. Plasmin standard curves using Novo, Kabi, and British standard plasmin.

AP (plasma) + PLI (excess) ⟶ AP.PLI + PLI

H-D-Val-Leu-Lys-pNA $\xrightarrow{PLI}$ H-D-Val-Leu-Lys-OH + pNA

Dil. plasma (1/30) in tris buffer pH 7.4 I 0.15	600 µl
Plasmin (0.25 CU/ml) in 50% glycerol + PEG	200 µl
incubate	
Substrate (3.5 mmol/l)	200 µl

FIG. 4. Principle of the method for α_2-antiplasmin determination.

ANTIPLASMIN ASSAY

The principle of the method is described in Fig. 4. It is of course important that the plasmin is free from any activator and we have also noticed that the Novo plasmin is not suitable, probably because of large amounts of lysine. As shown in Fig. 5 (lower curve), we found a very rapid initial inhibition of plasmin followed by a more progressive one (probably α_2-M). The upper curve which is usually

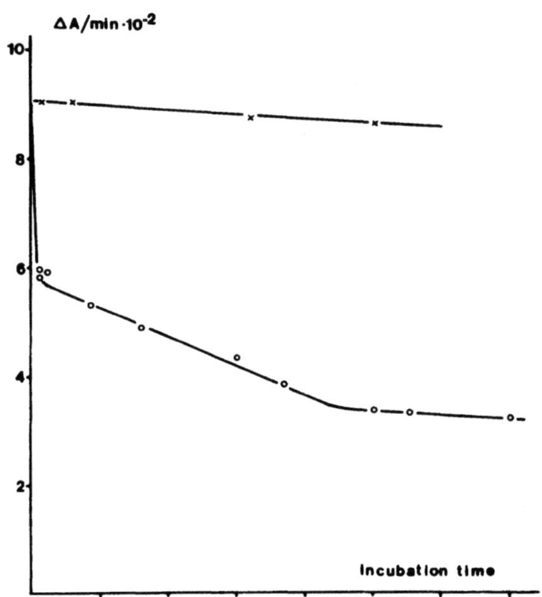

FIG. 5. Plasmin activity after different times of incubation in buffer (x) and plasma (o) diluted in buffer (n=2-3)

more horizontal represents only plasmin. The antiplasmin in question has been shown to be identical with the protein α_2-antiplasmin (3), which was discovered by three different research groups separately and for which the inhibition kinetics have been studied by two different groups. This inhibitor at first reacts very fast but reversibly with the lysine binding site of plasmin and then it binds irreversibly to the active site of the enzyme (7). According to the data in Fig. 6 (where the upper curve represents only plasmin and the lower curve plasmin + plasma), the amount of plasmin used may vary between certain limits. To obtain a large percental inhibition we have chosen a plasmin concentration of about 0.06 CU.

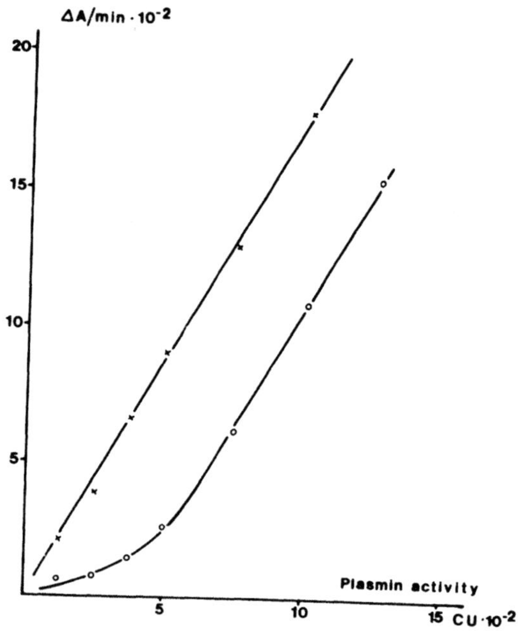

FIG. 6. Plasmin activity after incubation for 20 sec in buffer (x) and plasma (o) diluted in buffer. Different amounts of plasmin are used (n=2–3)

It has been suggested that even at short incubation times like 20 sec, other inhibitors like α_2-M may interfere (8). This would be the case especially at low α_2-antiplasmin and high α_2-M concentration.

Luckily enough, it was found possible to twist the method adding the substrate to the plasma dilution and the plasmin as last reagent which together with an initial rate measurement creates a very discriminating method (Note the possibility of automization with this single stage method!). However, using the two methods, no difference between the slopes using the initial rate technique (Fig. 7) was found and only a minor difference (ca 5% decrease) using the acetic acid stopped technique (Fig. 8). The twisted technique was in our hands not quite as reproducible as the earlier used technique.

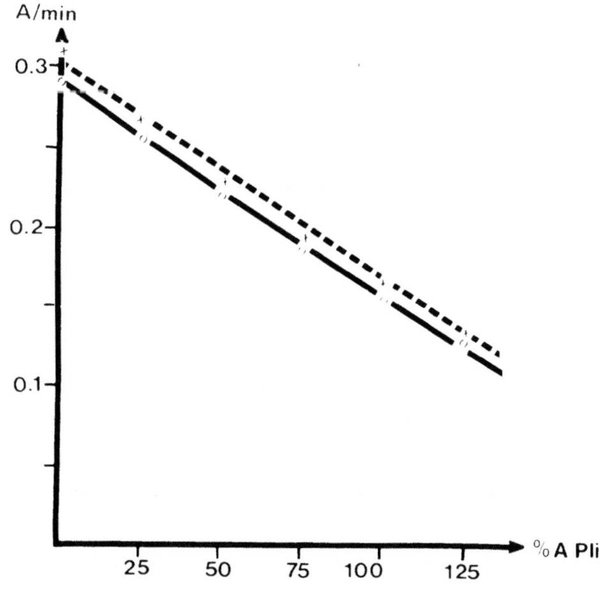

FIG. 7. Plasmin standard curves adding the substrate before (--x—) and after (-o-) the enzyme.

In stability tests on the antiplasmin kits (2 batches, 5 and 7 kits each), we found that after four weeks the plasmin activity had decreased by 8%. As the slopes of the standard curves decreased by the same percentage, it must be suspected that degraded plasmin consumes antiplasmin. This will, however, not interfere with the results of the assay because the sample is compared with a standard.

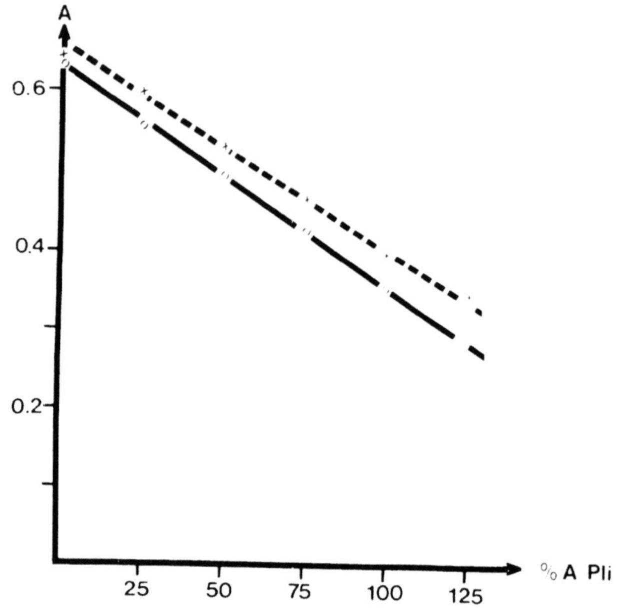

FIG. 8. Same as Fig. 7 but using the acid stopped method. 3 min incubation.

In the test series mentioned above, the reproducibility of the method was also determined. The slope and intercept of standard curves were calculated and the C.V. was about 3.5% for both. The day to day variation was about 3% and the kit to kit variation was about 2%.

Talking about antiplasmins, the possibility to assay α_2-M should be mentioned (9). If plasmin is added in excess to less diluted plasma and incubated for ca 5 min before Trasylol^R or SBTI is added to neutralize free plasmin, there will still be some activity left, viz plasmin-α_2-M complex which has 50-60% of the activity of free plasmin on S-2251. The reversibility of the plasmin-α_2-M complex has to be studied to optimize the method. Trypsin may also be used in a method for α_2-M determination.

PLASMINOGEN ASSAY

The principle of the method is shown in Fig. 9. SK was used in a molar excess compared to PLG (SK = Streptokinase, Kabikinase[R]). The pH and ionic strength optima for the two stages (activation and determination) have been optimized and pH 7.4 and ionic strength 0.05 was found suitable for both (2).

PLG (plasma) + SK ⟶ PLG.SK

H-D-Val-Leu-Lys-pNA $\xrightarrow{\text{PLG.SK}}$ H-D-Val-Leu-Lys-OH + pNA

Dil. plasma (1/40) in tris buffer pH 7.4 I 0.05	600 µl
SK (10,000 IU/ml)	200 µl
Incubate	
Substrate (3.0 mmol/l)	200 µl

FIG. 9. Principle of the method for plasminogen determination.

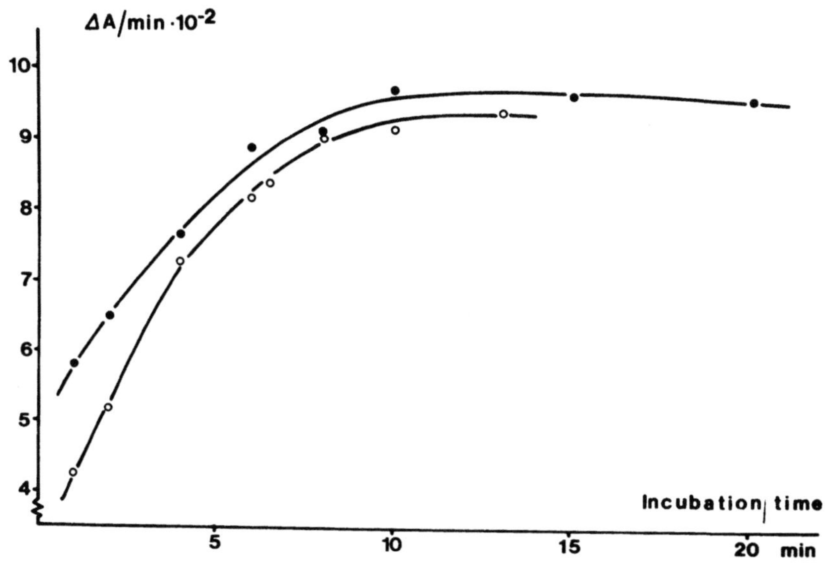

FIG. 10. PLG-SK activity after different times of incubation.
o = purified PLG. ● = normal human plasma.

As shown in Fig. 10, the incubation time (● = plasma, o = purified PLG) at 37°C should be 10 min. The fast initial rate of activation (50% after 1 min) and the longer time until full activity was reached may depend on a fast reaction between PLG and SK which is followed by a more time-consuming rearrangement of the complex. The difference in rate between the two steps in activation was increased by only decreasing the volume, but by increasing the temperature as well to 42°C the second step was speeded up considerably. At 42°C the activation was complete within 3 min.

The amount of SK needed for the activation was studied (Fig. 11) and found to be rather constant from 800-5,000 IU, activity decreasing slowly at higher or lower concentrations. 2,000 IU which is a molar excess of 40 times, is recommended. This would also allow for an anti-SK titer below 120,000 IU/ml of plasma $(\frac{2,000-800}{0.01})$. Suspecting higher anti-SK titers, 5,000 IU should be used allowing a titer of more than 400,000 IU. We have had reports that by using other brands of SK (e.g. the one from Behringwerke), the activity increased all the time with the amount of SK (10).

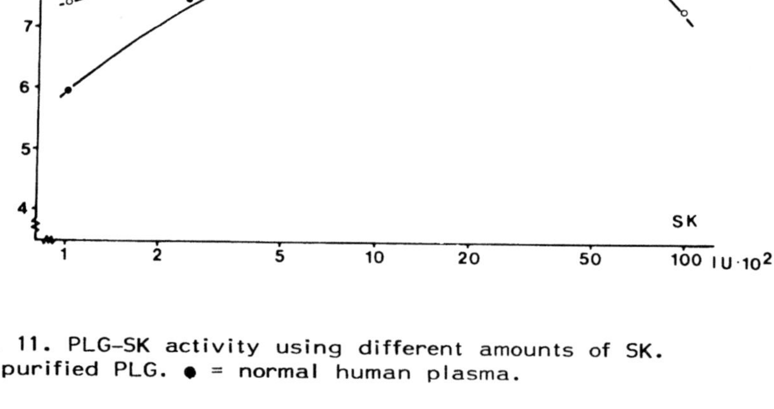

FIG. 11. PLG-SK activity using different amounts of SK. o = purified PLG. ● = normal human plasma.

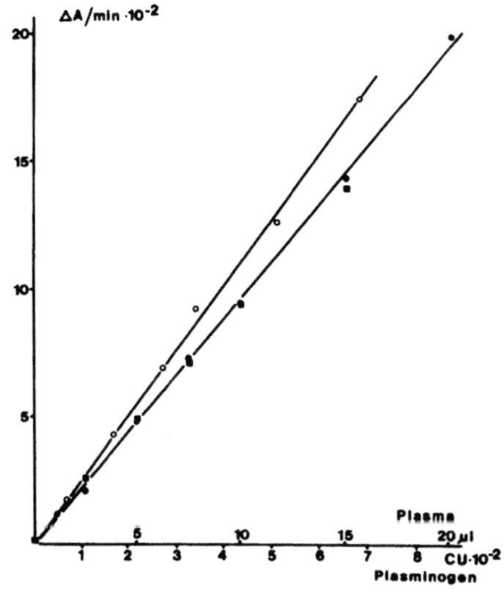

FIG. 12. Standard curves using different amounts of PLG (o) or plasma (•) or 20 µl of a mixture of normal plasma and PLG-free (adsorbed) plasma containing 100% of antiplasmin (■).

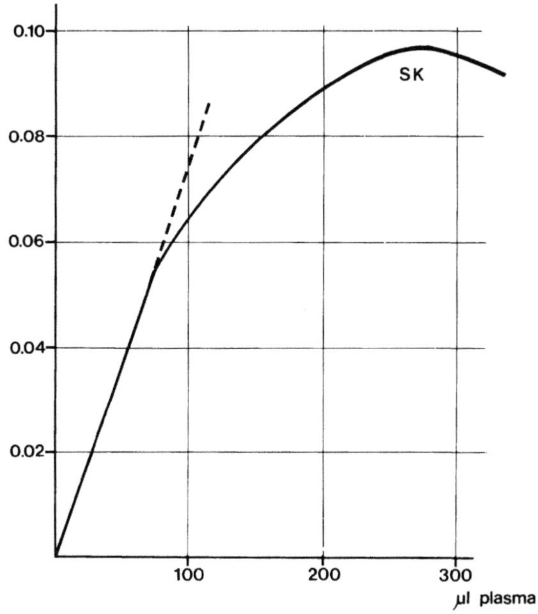

FIG. 13. Standard curve using different amounts of plasma.

The standard curves (Fig. 12) for purified PLG (o), diluted normal plasma (●), and normal plasma mixed with PLG deficient plasma (Lys-Sepharose, 100% antiplasmin (■)) are shown in this figure. The identity of the two latter curves with plasma containing different amounts of antiplasmin shows the absence of inhibition. The next figure (Fig. 13) shows a linear standard curve up to 80 µl (8 times recommended above) and at higher plasma concentrations there is probably a lack of SK (Data obtained with S-2160). The absence of inhibition (Fig. 14) was also proved by adding PLG deficient plasma to plasmin (lower curves, 2 different incubation times) and to SK activated PLG (upper curve).

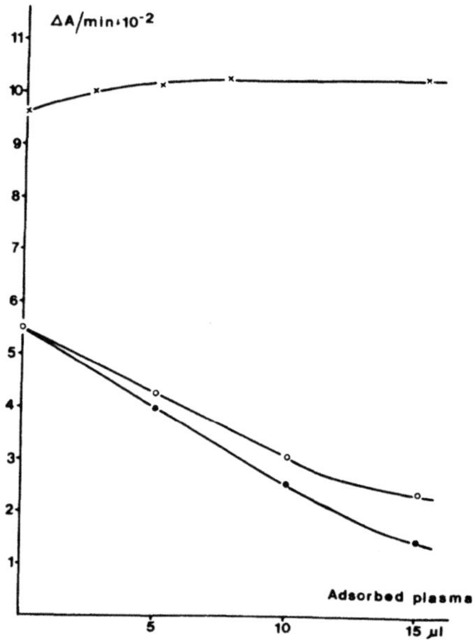

FIG. 14. Effect of different amounts of adsorbed plasma added to plasmin (incubation time 20 sec (o) and 5 min (●)) and PLG-SK (x, incubation time 10 min).

When using UK as an activator, the inhibition effect by plasma was evident.

When comparing approximately equimolar amounts of Glu-PLG, Lys-PLG, and plasmin in the method, it was found that the Lys-PLG-SK and plasmin-SK complexes gave 140% and 190% respectively compared to the native Glu-PLG-SK (4). At intermittent SK therapy, the amount of PLG in plasma should preferably be of samples taken before, not after the injection. In such a case plasmin may be inhibited by SBTI, but very preliminary studies with SBTI did not show a total inhibition of plasmin when SK was added after the inhibitor. When SBTI was added to PLG before SK, full activity was not obtained after 10 min incubation. This shows that further studies are needed.

If the PLG is acidified (which has been used to denaturate inhibitors), the activity of the complex is increased considerably (11). As this cannot be an effect caused by the destruction of inhibitors, it must depend on some conformational changes in the PLG molecule and we have observed similar effects with purified PLG. When PLG levels below 20% are expected, e.g. during SK treatment, the amount of plasma should be increased to obtain a higher activity.

STREPTOKINASE STANDARDIZATION

The method suggested is shown in Fig. 15.

SK + PLG (excess) $\longrightarrow$ Plasmin

H-D-Val-Leu-Lys-pNA $\xrightarrow{\text{Plasmin}}$ H-D-Val-Leu-Lys-OH + pNA

Tris buffer pH 7.4, I 0.05	300 µl
PLG 2.5 CU/ml, pH 3-4	100 µl
SK (50-600 IU/ml), 0.5% PEG	100 µl
Incubate (2 min)	
Substrate 3 mM + buffer 1 + 4	2,000 µl
Mix and read ΔA/min on a recorder	

FIG. 15. Principle of the method for streptokinase standardization.

The molar excess of PLG is at least 5 times.

By using different amounts of PLG as a substrate a K_m = 0.26 CU/ml was found (4). This figure is two potencies of ten lower than the figure obtained for UK (12). The PLG concentration in the first stage is $2.K_m$ and less than 20% of it is consumed in the method. By adding a relatively large volume before measuring the plasmin activity, a constant reaction rate with the substrate was obtained. A standard curve is shown in Fig. 16. It was approximately linear from 5 to 50 IU of SK. The slope decreases at higher concentrations, probably because of lack of PLG; S.D. ± 1 IU from 5-50 IU (n=5 for each concentration).

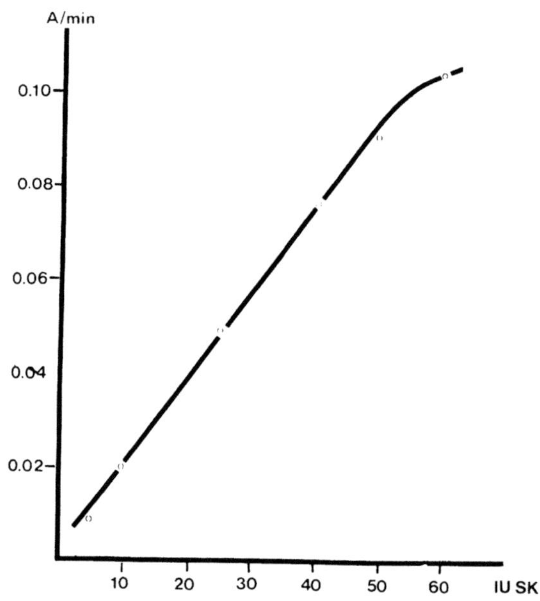

FIG. 16. Standard curve using different amounts of SK and a constant PLG concentration.

STANDARDIZATION OF PROTEOLYTIC PLASMINOGEN ACTIVATORS

For PLG activators like UK and tissue activators (TA) chromogenic substrates as well as standardization methods have already been developed. However, these activities should be compared with their activity as PLG activators. Such a technique may also increase the sensitivity because PLG acts as a multiplier.

Urokinase has been measured in this way using low concentrations of EACA, purified PLG and S-2251 (Whur P. Personal communications) (13).

Concerning TA, fibrin has probably some importance for its activation capacity but we cannot yet report on any successful method for its determination.

Another plasminogen activator that might be of some importance in the so-called intrinsic activation of plasminogen is kallikrein. Methods for the determination of plasma prekallikrein and kallikrein inhibitors in plasma using chromogenic substrates have been proposed (14,15).

To determine activator inhibitors, substrates for the different activators would be an important tool. This has been studied by Gallimore (16).

DETERMINATION OF ACTIVITY IN PLASMA

We will just briefly mention this subject. Partly because others like Professors Latallo and Duckert have done a lot of interesting work on this.

Proteolytc activities in plasma on the substrate S-2251 are expected from three different sources. Mainly plasmin-α_2-M complex will be found but under certain circumstances plasmin (which might be inhibited by SBTI or Trasylol) and PLG-SK or plasmin-SK activities (which might be inhibited by Trasylol) may be found (By using these inhibitors, it might be possible to determine SK in plasma).

Studying these factors, the occasion of blood sampling, treatment of sample, and speed of analysis will probably be critical because the fibrinolytic system may be in a rather dynamic state.

SUGGESTIONS FOR FUTURE DEVELOPMENTS

Besides some suggestions of new methods proposed above, we would like to add the following :

1. It would be of great value if somebody could do some further studies of the effect of different plasmins on different substrates.
2. A chromogenic substrate method for titration of the SK antibodies might be of interest.
3. Studies on proteolytic activities in plasma are important.
4. A chromogenic substrate method for the determination of α_2-M should be established.

TABLE 4

CHROMOGENIC SUBSTRATE METHODS WITHIN THE FIBRINOLYTIC SYSTEM

SUBSTRATE	METHOD	COMMENT
S-2251	Plasminogen in plasma	Lab instr
"	α_2-antiplasmin in plasma	Lab instr
"	α_2-macroglobulin in plasma	Proposed method
"	Plasmin-like activity in plasma	e g α_2-M complex
"	Streptokinase standardization	Prel method
"	Streptokinase determination in plasma	-
"	Activator activity in plasma	Possible screening method
"	Antistreptokinase titer	-
"	Urokinase/Tissue activator standardization	Proposed method
S-2444	Urokinase standardization	Lab instr
"	Urokinase in plasma	Proposed method
"	Urokinase inhibitor in plasma	Proposed method
S-2322 or similar	Tissue activator standardization	Prel method
"	Activator in tissues	Proposed method
"	Activator inhibitor in plasma	-
S-2302	Prekallikrein in plasma	Lab instr
"	Prekallikrein activator activity in plasma	-
"	Kallikrein inhibitor in plasma	Proposed method

5. Studies on the parallelism between chromogenic substrate- and PLG-splitting activities of different proteolytic PLG activators ought to be performed. Preferably by those preparing these enzymes.
6. General clinical studies are, as far as we understand, important in two fields : a) monitoring of fibrinolytic treatment, b) study of the importance of fibrinolytic factor levels in connection with hypercoagulability and thrombosis (Possibly also in connection with bleeding complications and DIC).
7. Connections between contact activation of the plasma kinin system and the intrinsic fibrinolysis activation may also be further studied using chromogenic substrates.

To sum up, we would like to present a table of existing and possible methods in, or connected to, the fibrinolytic system (Table 4).

REFERENCES

1. Friberger P, Knös M, Gustavsson S, Aurell L, and Claeson G. 1979. A new specific substrate for the determination of plasmin activity. In : Chromogenic Peptide Substrates, Scully MF and Kakkar VV (Eds), Churchill Livingstone, pp 121-127.
2. Friberger P and Knös M. 1979. Plasminogen determination in human plasma. In : Chromogenic Peptide Substrates, Scully MF and Kakkar VV (Eds), Churchill Livingstone, pp 128-139.
3. Teger-Nilsson AC, Friberger P, and Gyzander E. 1977. Determination of a new rapid plasmin inhibitor in human blood by means of a plasmin specific tripeptide substrate. Scand.J.Clin.Lab.Invest. 37, 403-404.
4. Knös M and Friberger P. 1979. Methods for plasminigen determination in human plasma and for streptokinase standardization. In : Progress in Chemical Fibrinolyis and Thrombolysis Vol IV, Davidson JF (Ed), Churchill Livingstone, pp 154-158.
5. Claeson G, Aurell L, Karlsson G, Gustavsson S, Friberger P, Arielly S, and Simonsson R. 1979. Design of chromogenic peptide substrates. In : Chromogenic Peptide Substrates, Scully MF and Kakkar VV (Eds), Churchill Livingstone, pp 20-30.
6. Friberger P, Claeson G, Knös M, Aurell L, Arielly S, and Simonsson R. 1979. Activity of plasminogen ativators on tripeptide chromogenic substrates. In : Progress in Chemical Fibrinolysis and Thrombolysis Vol IV, Davidson JF (Ed), Churchill Livingstone, pp 149-153.
7. Collen D and Wiman B. 1979. The fast-acting plasmin inhibitor of human plasma. The Prix Servier Lecture. In : Progress in Chemical Fibrinolysis and Thrombolysis Vol IV, Davidson JF (Ed), Churchill Livingstone, pp 11-19.
8. Friberger P. 1979. Discussion in Chromogenic Peptide Substrates, Scully MF and Kakkar VV (Eds), Churchill Livingstone, pp 246.
9. Latallo ZS, Teisseyre E, and Lopaciuk S. 1979. Evaluation of a fibrinolytic profile of plasma using chromogenic substrates. In : Chromogenic Peptide Substrates, Scully MF and Kakkar VV (Eds), Churchill Livingstone, pp 262-266.

10. Korsan-Bengtsen K, Johnsen M, and Gustavsson G. 1977. Evidence for the presence in human plasma of a streptokinase co-factor separable from plasminogen. Thrombos.Haemostas. 38, 135.
11. Latallo ZS. 1979. Discussion in Chromogenic Peptide Substrates, Scully MF and Kakkar VV (Eds), Churchill Livingstone, pp 139.
12. Gaffney PJ and Philo R. 1979. Comparison of bioassays and assays using chromogenic substrates. An interim report. Paper presented at the meeting on "Synthetic Substrates and Inhibitors", organized by the Subcommittee on Synthetic Substrates and Inhibitors, London, July 14th, 1979.
13. Whur P. Personal Communications.
14. Friberger P, Eriksson E, Gustavsson S, and Claeson G. 1979. Determination of prekallikrein in plasma by means of a chromogenic tripeptide substrate for plasma kallikrein. In Kinins-II, Fujii S et al (Eds), Plenum Publishing Corporation, pp 67-82.
15. Gallimore MJ, Amundsen E, Larsbraaten M, Lyngaas K, and Fareid E. 1979. Studies on plasma inhibitors of plasma kallikrein using chromogenic peptide substrate assays. Thromb.Res. 16, 695-703.
16. Gallimore MJ. 1979. Inhibitors of plasminogen activation present in human plasma. In : The Physiological Inhibitors of Coagulation and Fibrinolysis, Collen D, Wiman B, and Verstraete M (Eds), Elsevier/North-Holland Biomedical Press, pp 199-217.

α_2-ANTIPLASMIN ASSAY : AMIDOLYTIC AND IMMUNOLOGICAL METHOD. CRITICAL EVALUATION. RESULTS IN A CLINICAL MATERIAL.

M. SAMAMA, N. SCHLEGEL*, B. CAZENAVE, M.H. HORELLOU, J. CONARD, M. CASTEL and R. DOUENIAS*.

Laboratoire Central d'Hématologie, Hôtel-Dieu, 75181 Paris Cédex 04, and *Laboratoire Central d'Hématologie et d'Immunologie, Hôpital Bretonneau, 75018 Paris, France.

Recently a new and physiologically important inhibitor of plasmin has been identified in human plasma (1-3).

This fast acting plasmin inhibitor has been called α_2-antiplasmin or α_2-plasmin inhibitor. Identification and physiological properties of this inhibitor are summarized in Table 1.

TABLE 1.

α_2-Antiplasmin characteristics.

- M.W. = 70,000 - SYNTHESIS IN THE LIVER.
- SINGLE CHAIN GLYCOPROTEIN (CARBOHYDRATE 13%)
- REACTS WITH THE LIGHT (B) CHAIN OF PLASMIN
  ⟶ STOICHIOMETRIC COMPLEX (M.W. = 150,000)
- PLASMA CONCENTRATION : 1 μM - 1.5 μM (7 MG%)
- PLASMA HALF LIFE 2.6 ± 0.3 DAYS.
- WEAK ACUTE PHASE REACTANT PROTEIN
- CONGENITAL DEFICIENCY = MIYASATO DISEASE.

α_2-Antiplasmin can be evaluated in human plasma with an amidolytic method using a chromogenic substrate : Kabi S-2251 (4,5) or with the Laurell method using a specific antiserum[1].

The correlation between these two methods is very satisfactory in most patients who were not receiving any thrombolytic therapy (r=0.67).

However, the specificity of both methods is not restricted to α_2-antiplasmin. Firstly a part of α_2-antiplasmin is not active or is denaturated. After addition of increasing concentrations of urokinase, α_2-antiplasmin evaluated by the amidolytic method decreases to zero, while some free α_2-antiplasmin, as shown by crossed immunoelectrophoresis is still persistent (Table 2). Similar results are obtained after plasminogen addition to plasma in order to increase plasmin formation (Table 3.).

TABLE 2.

Evolution of α_2-antiplasmin activity and α_2-antiplasmin antigen during plasminogen activation in vitro in human plasma.

UK concentration I.U.	α_2-Antiplasmin amidolytic method	Crossed immunoelectrophoresis
0	95%	1 peak
100	28%	2 peaks
200	22%	2 peaks
300	7%	2 peaks
400	0%	2 peaks

TABLE 3.

Evolution of α_2-antiplasmin activity and α_2-antiplasmin antigen. Plasminogen activation in vitro in human plasma enriched with human plasminogen.

UK concentration I.U.	Human plasminogen added 30 mg% F.C.	α_2-antiplasmin amidolytic method S-2251	Crossed immunoelectrophoresis
0	0	90%	1 peak
0	+	65%	2 peaks
100	0	37%	2 peaks
100	+	0%	2 peaks
200	0	10%	2 peaks
200	+	0%	2 peaks
300	0	0%	2 peaks
300	+	0%	2 peaks

In parallel it is well known that plasmin-α_2-macroglobulin complex is active on the synthetic substrate. In contrast plasmin-Kunitz inhibitor complex is not active, as shown in Figure 1.

Using crossed immunoelectrophoresis we have noticed that in the presence of a high concentration of Kunitz inhibitor a competitive reaction between α_2-antiplasmin and Kunitz inhibitor directed against plasmin can be suspected.

[1] Obtained as a generous gift from Dr. Collen (Leuven).

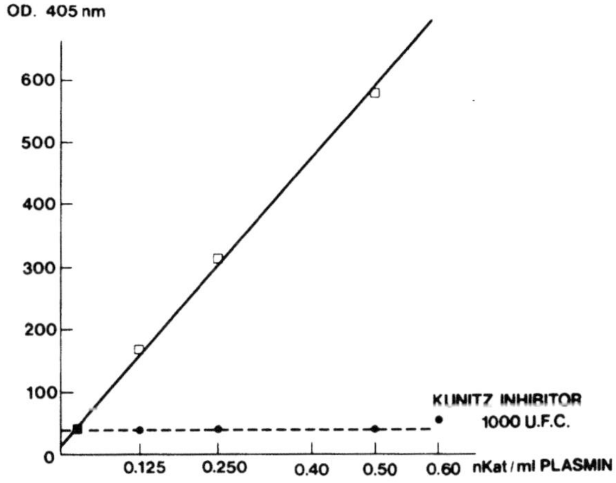

FIG. 1. Inhibition of purified plasmin by Kunitz inhibitor. Plasmin + buffer (□), plasmin + Kunitz inhibitor (●).

The results about the specificity of the immunological and the amidolytic method are summarized in Table 4.

TABLE 4.
Specificity of the methods used for α_2-antiplasmin determination.

	Laurell method	Crossed immuno-electrophoresis	Amidolytic method S-2251
Free α_2-antiplasmin	+	+	+
Plasmin-α_2-antiplasmin complex	+	+	0
Plasmin-α_2-M complex	0	0	+

We have evaluated α_2-antiplasmin in clinical material, and especially in patients with cirrhosis, disseminated intravascular coagulation (DIC) and patients treated with thrombolytic or defibrinating agents.

The main results are summarized in Table 5. No modification is observed in patients with antecedents of deep venous thrombosis (DVT). The α_2-antiplasmin level is increased in Behçet disease, which is an original finding.

TABLE 5.
α_2-Antiplasmin in clinical material.

	N	Mean	Range
Control	33	97.9%	80 to 130%
Pregnant women	12	108.2%	90 to 120%
Acute DVT	5	113.0%	85 to 120%
Recurrent DVT	22	104.0%	65 to 120%
Behçet disease	8	140.6%	125 to 200%

In contrast in 24 cirrhotic patients we have noticed an important decrease in α_2-antiplasmin which is correlated with the prolongation of the thromboplastin time (r = 0.55). The mean level is very similar in patients with normal or increased FDP. Thus, the decrease in α_2-antiplasmin seems to be due to insufficient liver synthesis and/or to DIC (Table 6).

TABLE 6.
α_2-Antiplasmin in liver cirrhosis (24 cases).

Fibrinogen level below 300 mg/dl	
Increased FDP	Normal FDP
14 patients	10 patients
Mean : 35%	Mean : 37%
Range : 15 to 45%	Range : 17 to 60%

We have also studied the plasma α_2-antiplasmin level in 25 patients with acute, subacute or chronic compensated or uncompensated disseminated intravascular coagulation (DIC) (Table 7). In compensated DIC with elevated FDP but normal fibrinogen level, the α_2-antiplasmin is higher than in uncompensated DIC : consequently, this test may be an additional tool for the diagnosis of DIC.

TABLE 7.

α_2-Antiplasmin in DIC (25 cases).

		Increased FDP	
		Fg ↘	Fg normal
Promyelocytic leukemia	7		
Acute myeloblastic leukemia	6		
Cancer + metastasis	6	m = 39%	m = 78%
Purpura fulminans	1	(15 to 73%)	(32 to 130%)
Dead foetus retention	1		
Ventricular aneurysm	2		
DIC during surgery	2	N = 18	N = 7

We have extended α_2-antiplasmin evaluation to SK or UK treated patients. At the doses administered, the decrease is more pronounced in SK than in UK-treated patients (Table 8). Moreover, the observed decrease in α_2-antiplasmin parallels the decrease in plasma fibrinogen.

TABLE 8.

α_2-Antiplasmin in SK- and UK-treated patients. Mean values and range observed after 24 hours of SK and 15 hours of UK.

	Fibrinogen	FDP	Plasminogen	α_2-Antiplasmin Laurell method
SK	70 mg/100 ml	179γ/ml	17%	17%
5 patients	(27 to 140)	(128 to 256)	(2 to 25)	(13 to 25)
UK	297 mg/100 ml	63γ/ml	65%	46%
20 patients	(100 to 500)	(1 to 256)	(25 to 100)	(15 to 84)

SK : 150,000 I.U./hour
UK : 2,000 CTA units/kg/hour

In defibrase treated patients, a decrease in α_2-antiplasmin is also found at any time during treatment. Crossed immunoelectrophoresis performed in these patients clearly demonstrates the presence of plasmin-α_2-antiplasmin complex in the plasma (6).

In conclusion, α_2-plasmin inhibitor evaluation with immunological and amidolytic method is a useful test, reproducible and usually reliable although its specificity must be questioned in some cases.

This test could be very useful in patients with liver disease and in DIC, especially if it is a compensated DIC. In these last cases, α_2-antiplasmin can be a very useful diagnostic tool.

SUMMARY

α_2-Antiplasmin has been studied in a clinical material by two methods : amidolytic and immunological. A good correlation is observed between these two methods, although the specificity of each method must be questioned in some cases.

An important decrease was noticed in cirrhotic patients, in patients with compensated or uncompensated disseminated intravascular coagulation, and in SK- or UK-treated patients.

At the doses administered, the decrease is more pronounced in SK-treated patients and parallels the decrease in the fibrinogen level. In defibrase-treated patients a decrease in α_2-antiplasmin is also found at any time of treatment and crossed immunoelectrophoresis performed in these patients clearly demonstrates the presence of plasmin-α_2-antiplasmin complex in the plasma.

The α_2-antiplasmin evaluation may be a useful tool for the diagnosis of DIC, especially in compensated states and during thrombolytic treatment.

REFERENCES

1. Collen D. 1976. Identification and some properties of a new fast-reacting plasmin inhibitor in human plasma. Eur.J.Biochem. 69, 209-216.
2. Moroi M and Aoki N. 1976. Isolation and characterization of alpha 2 plasmin inhibitor from human plasma. A novel proteinase inhibitor which inhibits activator induced clot lysis. J.Biol.Chem. 251,5956-5965.
3. Müllertz S and Clemmensen I. 1976. The primary inhibitor of plasmin in human plasma. Biochem.J. 159, 545-553.
4. Edy J, Collen D, and Verstraete M. 1978. Quantitation of the plasma protease inhibitor antiplasmin with the chromogenic substrate S-2251. In : Progress in Chemical Fibrinolysis and Thrombolysis Vol 3, Davidson JF, Rowan RM, Samama MM, and Desnoyers PC (Eds), Raven Press, New York, pp 315-322.
5. Teger-Nilsson AC, Friberger P, and Gyzander E. 1977. Determination of a new rapid plasmin inhibitor in human blood by means of a plasmin specific tripeptide substrate. Scand.J.Clin.Lab.Invest. 37, 403-404.
6. Samama M, Conard J, Cazenave B, Derlon A, Gaudric A, and Coscas, G. 1979. Modification of α_2-plasmin inhibitor during treatments by a defibrinating agent. Thrombos.Haemostas. 42, 277.

DISCUSSION

J.W. ten Cate : We have used a similar method and obtained similar results. The problem is to know what the therapeutical consequences are at low levels of α_2-antiplasmin in patients with DIC.

M. Samama : It seems that patients with very low α_2-antiplasmin levels are those with a very severe consumption coagulopathy and severe bleeding. We have treated a few cases by infusion of fresh frozen plasma.

D. Collen : At the clinical level the α_2-antiplasmin assay is mostly a research tool at the moment. Do you think it might have an application in the control of thrombolytic therapy?

M. Samama : We have not enough data to say this at the moment. It seems that in patients there is a very good correlation between an important fibrinogen decrease and α_2-antiplasmin decrease. It seems that α_2-antiplasmin protects fibrinogen. In our opinion, for streptokinase therapy α_2-antiplasmin evaluation would be an indirect indication of the effect of the treatment and maybe this would show a good correlation with the regimen used by Duckert and his group. They infuse plasmin to saturate α_2-antiplasmin and then they infuse streptokinase. But I don't think we have enough evidence for this assessment. We can say that during urokinase therapy with doses that are used in our country the level of α_2-antiplasmin is less depressed than during streptokinase therapy. This might mean that urokinase treatment is less active, but this is only hypothetical.

G. Wijngaards : In one of your slides you showed that in Behçet's disease there was an increased level of α_2-antiplasmin as determined immunologically by the Laurell method. We have done similar studies and observed in a severe case an increased plasmin inhibition of the slow type. Have you done a functional assay of the α_2-antiplasmin in these plasmas?

M. Samama : No, we have not. But it would be interesting to do it because we have a study in progress in Behçet's disease with the cuff test and α_2-antiplasmin evaluation. I think we will do it.

R. Lijnen : Since part of our α_2-antiplasmin seems to be inactive towards plasmin, can you then expect to find a good correlation between an amidolytic and an immunological assay?

M. Samama : We found a good correlation between the 2 methods. The lower value obtained with the Laurell method was 15% in a patient during streptokinase treatment; with the chromogenic assay we found in this patient less than 5% of α_2-antiplasmin. But still the correlation between both methods is satisfactory.

D. Collen : I think that the inactive α_2-antiplasmin in plasma actually is inactivated during activation of the fibrinolytic system. We have some data suggesting that it is a side product of the plasmin-α_2-antiplasmin reaction; you only see it in activated samples. If you isolate the α_2-antiplasmin it reacts in a purified system with plasmin in a stoichiometric reaction with 100% yield.

Cl. Bouvier : The more we discuss about clotting enzymes and inhibitors, the more it should be stressed that we are not so much interested in the presence of the antigen, as we are to know if it is active or not; for factor XIII for instance.

D. Collen : There are at present only 2 families described with a congenital deficiency, this is absence of antigen and activity. Maybe sooner or later a defective molecule will be found.

Unidentified discussant : Do you think the α_2-antiplasmin assay will be of practical value in the future?

M. Samama : Together with a hepatologist we are now doing a study in a group of 35 patients with liver disease where all the tests are performed and we are doing an α_2-antiplasmin determination as well. We will try to find out if it has any practical value. At the moment we can only say that the level is depressed in patients with liver disease.

L.H. Kahlé : I think that often the AT III level will correlate with α_2-antiplasmin.

D. Collen : Indeed, it correlates quite well.

L.H. Kahlé : We had several patients with low AT III levels and only slightly decreased levels of α_2-antiplasmin; in more severe liver cirrhosis the α_2-antiplasmin is decreased also. Probably you can detect the development of cirrhosis by using both methods.

EXPERIENCES WITH THE DETERMINATION OF KALLIKREIN, PLASMINOGEN AND ANTIPLASMIN USING CHROMOGENIC SUBSTRATES:CLINICAL APPLICATION

H.H.D.M. VAN VLIET

University Hospital Dijkzigt, Department of Hematology, Rotterdam, The Netherlands.

INTRODUCTION

The development and availability of chromogenic substrates is very promising because they offer the possibility to determine parameters of coagulation and fibrinolysis by means of an automated enzyme analyzer. Especially for the laborious (and time consuming) determinations of fibrinolytic activities this development is very attractive and makes these determinations accessible for less specialized laboratories.

In various diseases, summarised in Table 1, measurement of fibrinolysis has diagnostic value. Determinations are particularly important in cases of DIC, but also to detect deficiencies of the enzymes involved in fibrinolysis as possible causes of thrombosis or hemorrhagic diathesis. We have studied especially subjects with relapsing idiopathic thromboses. Theoretically one may assume that a lowering of fibrinolytic activity, c.q. by a decrease of fibrinolytic enzymes (activators) or an increase of inhibitors, will enhance the risk of thrombosis, whereas increased fibrinolysis may cause a hemorrhagic diathesis.

The activation mechanism of intrinsic fibrinolysis is shown in Figure 1. The enzymes/inhibitors which can be determined at present with the chromogenic substrates and methods are underlined. This includes the determinations of concentration, activitation and effect of fibrinolytic inhibitors, like the activator of prekallikrein, the concentration of plasminogen and inhibitors of plasmin. Routinely in most laboratories fibrinolysis is measured by determination of fibrinogen, FDP and fibrin monomers in plasma, and fibrinolytic activity is determined by the fibrin plate method or the lysis of clotted euglobulin proteins, whole blood or diluted blood. However, these determinations have serious disadvantages because they are laborious, insensitive,

TABLE 1.

Various disorders in which assessment of fibrinolysis has diagnostic value.

Primary disorders of fibrinolysis:	congenital deficiencies of plasminogen, antiplasmin, fibrinolytic activators.
Secondary (reactive) disorders:	liver disease prostatic carcinoma amniotic fluid embolism disseminated intravascular coagulation sepsis acute leukemia surgical procedures vasculitis : Behçet's disease solution of the placenta

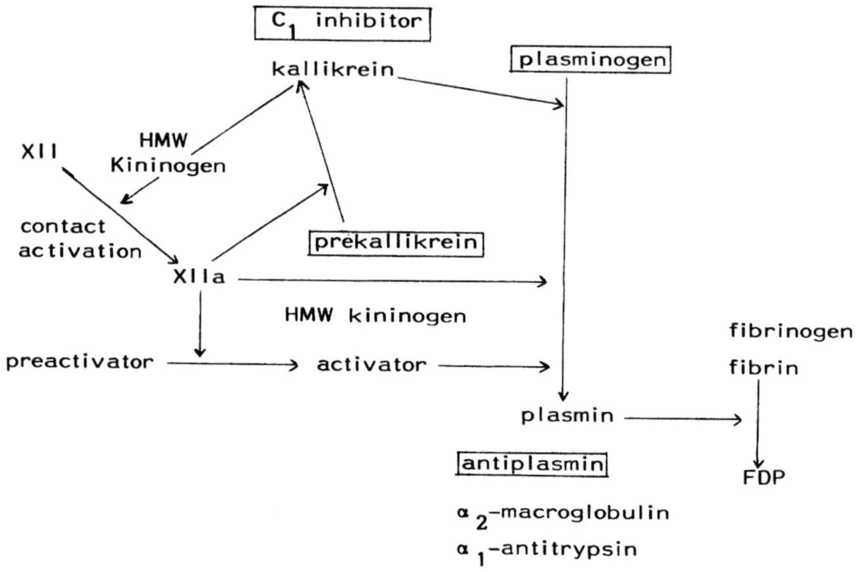

FIG. 1. Activation mechanism of intrinsic fibrinolysis.

poorly reproducible, time consuming and, as mentioned before, unsuitable for automation. Determinations with the aid of chromogenic substrates do not have these disadvantages.

The principles of the determination methods are outlined in Figure 2. The necessary specificity is obtained by specific activation methods and by the structure of the synthetic substrates.

<u>Plasminogen/plasmin determination</u>

Plasminogen (plasma) —(streptokinase)→ plasmin

plasmin + Chromogenic substrate S-2251/chromozym PL → p-nitroaniline

<u>Antiplasmin determination</u>

Excess plasmin + plasma (antiplasmin) → plasmin-inhibitor complex

Chromogenic substrate S-2251/chromozym PL —(residual plasmin)→ p-nitroaniline

<u>Prekallikrein/kallikrein determination</u>

prekallikrein (plasma) + dextran sulphate cephotest —(4°C)→ kallikrein

kallikrein + Chromogenic substrate S-2302/chromozym PK → p-nitroaniline

FIG. 2. Principles of the methods.

RESULTS

In a group of patients with bronchial carcinoma, prekallikrein levels were determined. According to the literature a small increase in fibrinogen turnover can be observed in these patients, as an indication of a low grade DIC. The usual plasma coagulation/fibrinolysis determinations did not show decreased concentrations of the different factors.

The results did show a very small decrease in average prekallikrein content to 80% of normal. However, the activation of prekallikrein to kallikrein turned out to be significantly decreased. The frequency distribution demonstrates that 76% of the patients had a decreased activation of less than 50% of standard (Figure 3). The cause of this decrease is still under investigation, but the preliminary results suggest that the determination of prekallikrein/kallikrein activation is a sensitive tool to establish low grade DIC, which is not noticed by the usual plasma coagulation/fibrinolysis measurements.

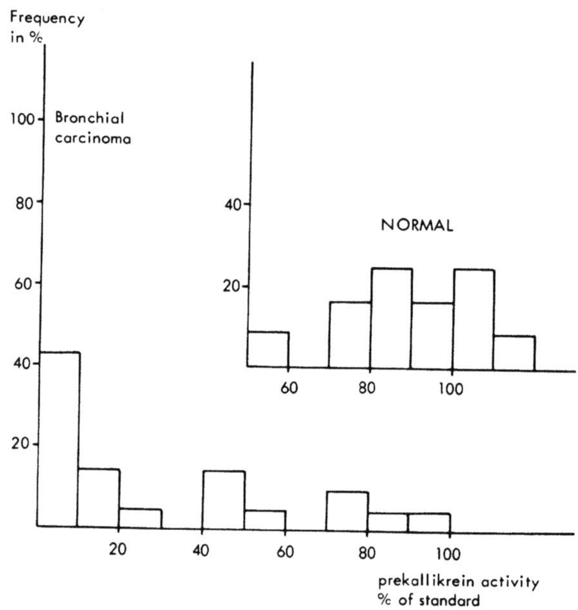

FIG. 3. Frequency distribution of activation activity of prekallikrein in plasma of patients with bronchial carcinoma.

Furthermore follow up studies were done in patients with different causes of DIC by determining the fibrinolytic parameters, the plasminogen and antiplasmin concentrations, together with antithrombin III.

The follow up of one patient with severe liver insufficiency is demonstrated in Figure 4. The concentrations of factor I, V and the vitamin K-dependent factors are very low and also because of insufficient hepatic synthesis, the plasminogen, antiplasmin and AT III plasma contents were diminished. Temporary elevation of the concen-

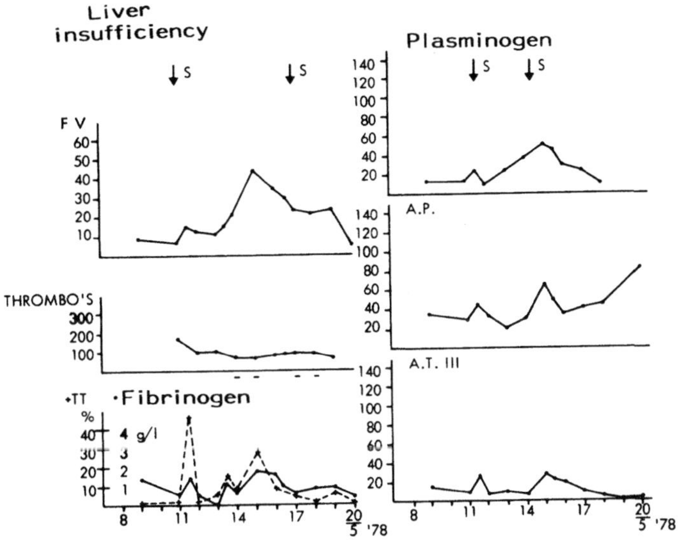

FIG. 4. Follow up of plasminogen, antiplasmin and AT III plasma concentrations during liver cirrhosis. Plasma was substituted at indicated time intervals (S).

tration of these factors was the result of plasma replacement therapy. Low grade chronic DIC was studied in a subject with an adenocarcinoma of the prostate (Figure 5). DIC was suspected because of measurable FDP and a small decrease of AT III. Accordingly, the concentration of antiplasmin was also decreased, whereas the plasminogen concentration was not reduced. As shown, the administration of heparin had only a small effect on both the antiplasmin and AT III concentration, which made FDP formation by thrombin generation questionable.

A gynaecological patient with pre-eclampsia was studied before and after parturition (Figure 6). Pre-delivery indications for DIC were a low platelet count, the presence of FDP and a lowered fibrinogen concentration. The AT III content was decreased, the plasminogen concentration was normal, but activated fibrinolysis could be demonstrated by a low antiplasmin level. During low-dose heparin therapy both AT III and antiplasmin concentrations decreased. Shortly after parturition the measurable AT Iil concentration dropped to only 20% of normal but this AT III and antiplasmin rose to normal levels. Remarkable

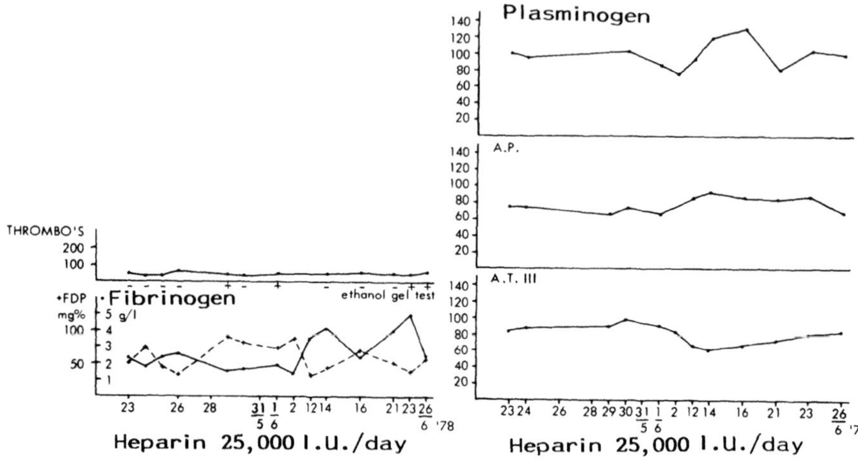

FIG. 5. Carcinoma of the prostate with intravascular coagulation.

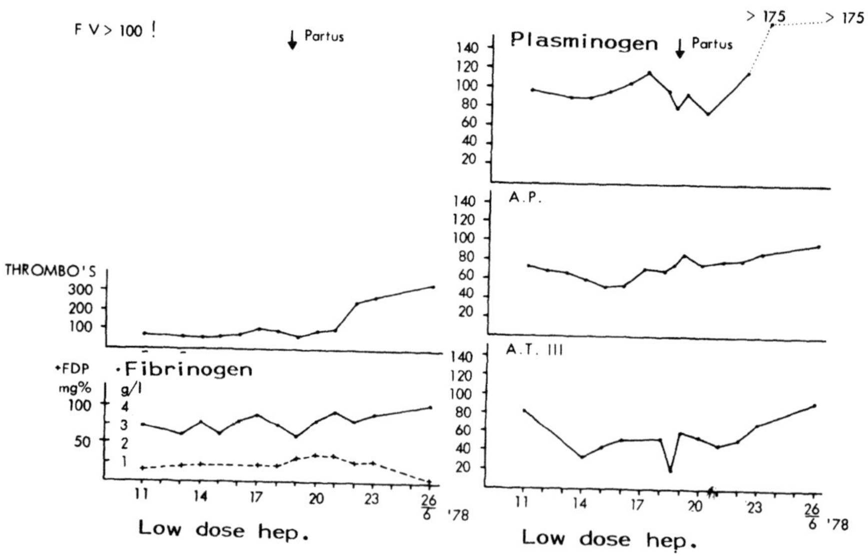

FIG. 6. Plasminogen, antiplasmin and AT III concentration in plasma pre- and post-partum by a patient with pre-eclampsia.

is the almost doubling of the plasminogen concentration, which however may be normal during the post-partum period, because this was noticed also in the following two patients, who had acute DIC, caused in one by intrauterine trauma and in the other by amniotic fluid embolism (Figures 7 and 8). Low fibrinogen and high FDP plasma concentrations were found, characteristic of DIC. However, the AT III concentrations were normal, which made DIC questionable as the underlying cause. The increased turnover of fibrinogen, evident from the low fibrinogen and high FDP value, may consequently not be the result of fibrinolysis but rather of fibrinogenolysis, as concluded from a decrease of the antiplasmin concentration. Normalisation was accompanied by an increase of fibrinogen and antiplasmin.

Acute DIC was also studied by a follow up of 3 patients with respectively meningococcal sepsis, multiple traumatic fractures and after an accidental infusion.

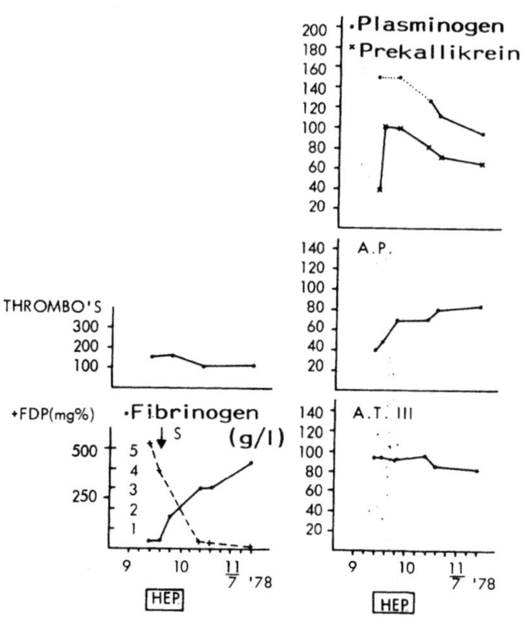

FIG. 7. Acute intravascular coagulation from intrauterine trauma, treated with heparin.

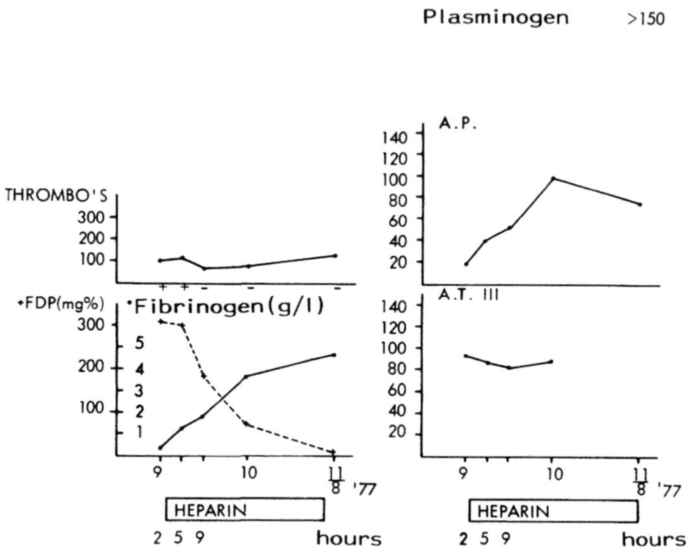

FIG. 8. Acute intravascular coagulation from amniotic fluid embolism, treated with heparin.

In contrast to the two pregnant women the AT III level in the latter three patients was decreased and remained low whereas the fibrinogen and antiplasmin values became normal. This discrepancy between a lasting decrease of AT III and a normalisation of antiplasmin seemed to be a poor prognostic sign of imminent circulatory complications (Figures 9, 10 and 11).

The last example illustrates the applicability during streptokinase treatment in a patient with pulmonary embolism (Figure 12). As a result of fibrinolytic activation by streptokinase, the plasminogen and fibrinogen concentration fell precinitously as did the inhibitor of fibrinolysis, antiplasmin. AT III shows a decrease to 60% of normal, probably as a result of coagulation activation induced by the therapy.

In conclusion our results demonstrate that the determinations of plasminogen, antiplasmin and AT III with the aid of chromogenic substrates form a valuable addition to the diagnostic determinations, which are presently available as an aid in the treatment of patients with coagulation/fibrinolytic complications.

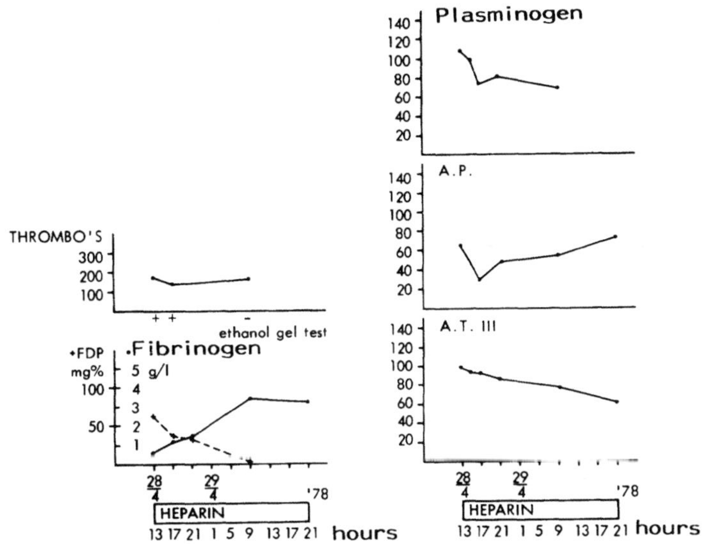

FIG. 9. Follow up of fibrinolytic parameters and antithrombin III during meningococcal sepsis. Patient was treated with heparin and substitution of different blood components.

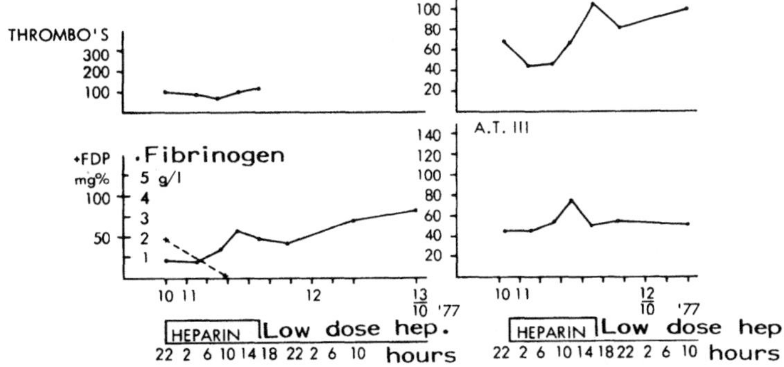

FIG. 10. Plasma concentrations of plasminogen, antiplasmin and AT III in a patient with multiple fractures, treated with heparin.

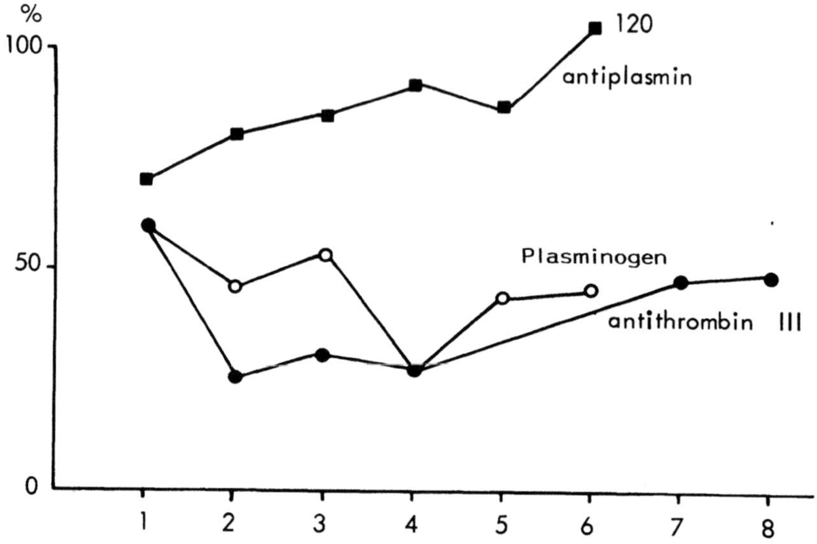

FIG. 11. Plasma concentrations of plasminogen, antiplasmin and AT III in a patient with DIC caused by an accidental infusion.

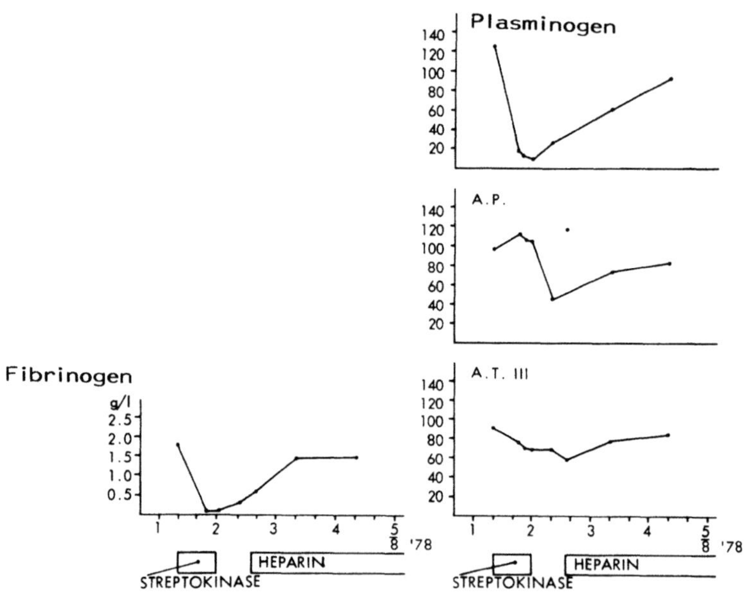

FIG. 12. Effect of plasmin on plasminogen and antiplasmin concentration during streptokinase therapy by pulmonary embolism.

NEW PROSPECTS IN THE ACTIVATION OF FIBRINOLYSIS

C. KLUFT

Gaubius Institute, Health Research Organization TNO, Herenstraat 5d, 2313 AD Leiden, The Netherlands.

INTRODUCTION

Blood clots are not permanent structures in the body. They only serve temporary functions : providing a haemostatic plug when haemorrhage occurs and forming a supporting medium during the subsequent repair process.

The blood clot and its matrix, fibrin, has to disappear again and its time of disappearance is of importance. Too rapid removal leads to renewed bleeding and interference with the tissue repair. Too late removal or persistence may lead to disorganization and tissue may grow out of shape.

Clots and fibrin can also be completely undesirable, as occurs in cases of thrombosis or diffuse intravascular coagulation; disappearance then has to be as rapid as possible to limit the damage.

The removal of fibrin clots (fibrinolysis) consequently needs to be a carefully regulated function in the body, which must be equipped to meet several challenges in haemostasis depending on the location and cause of the occurrence of fibrin clots.

This article deals with various routes of activation of the process of fibrinolysis.

FIBRINOLYSIS

During fibrinolysis the protein polymer fibrin is fragmented into soluble pieces (fibrin degradation products). The important proteolytic enzyme in this fragmentation is the serine protease plasmin.

Plasmin is not found free in the circulation, but must first be formed from a precursor, plasminogen, present in the blood. The conversion of plasminogen to plasmin is a process of limited proteolysis achieved by plasminogen activators (1). This process of activation of plasminogen and subsequent fibrinolysis is schematically presented in Figure 1.

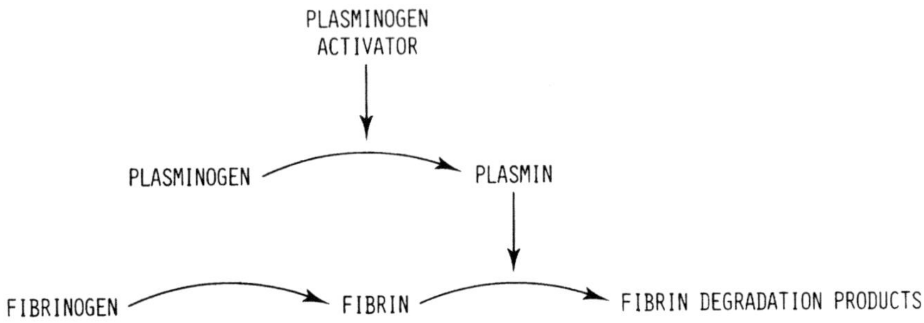

FIG. 1. Scheme for fibrinolysis

ACTIVATORS OF PLASMINOGEN

Plasminogen can be activated to plasmin by several plasminogen activators in the blood. These activators can be subdivided pragmatically into two groups, i.e. those of extrinsic and those of intrinsic origin.

The extrinsic plasminogen activator(s) found in the blood are released into the blood from tissue e.g. the vessel wall.

The intrinsic plasminogen activator(s) are generated from plasminogen proactivators circulating in the blood.

The occurrence of extrinsic or vascular activator activity in the blood has been known for a long time; the intrinsic plasminogen activator activity of the blood has only been appreciated in recent years. It is becoming increasingly evident that blood contains a complex intrinsic system of fibrinolysis activation, involving several plasminogen activators.

Extrinsic plasminogen activators

A very low level of extrinsic plasminogen activator can be continuously detected in the blood. Transient increases in this level can be observed after stimulated secretion of the extrinsic activator into the blood.

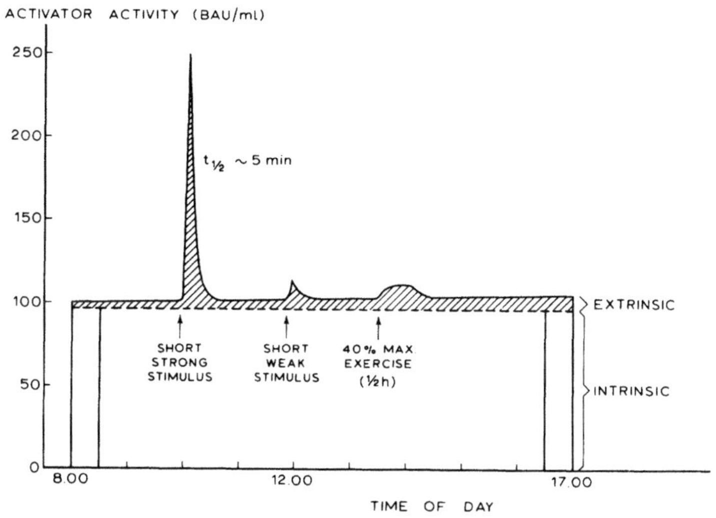

FIG. 2. Schematic representation of the plasma activator potential during daytime and after stimuli. The amount of activator activity is given in arbitrary blood activator units (BAU). See text for further description.

Changes in the plasma level of extrinsic activator and the effect of stimuli is schematically outlined in Figure 2. Early in the morning in a person at rest, the level is 1-2 blood activator units (BAU)/ml. At the end of the day, the level can be increased about two-fold; this is known as the diurnal increase in blood fibrinolytic activity (2). The mechanism of this diurnal rhythm is not yet understood.

Various stimuli can temporarily increase the blood level of extrinsic activator (reviewed by Astrup, 1977)(3), as shown in Figure 2 for three typical situations. The level can be dramatically increased by strong stimulation such as electric shock, injection of nicotinic acid or a short period of exhaustive exercise. Weaker stimuli such as stress or fright, adrenalin injection or moderate exercise give a smaller response (4).

As shown in the Figure, the plasma level of extrinsic activator increases following the stimulus, but decreases again rapidly after cessation of the stimulus. The disappearance of extrinsic activator from the circulation is mainly due to clearance by the liver (5), with an apparent half-life after exercise of about 5 minutes. In cases of liver disease, the clearance has been shown to be delayed.

The extrinsic system gives an impression of being a dynamic one which is able to react quickly and strongly to various stimuli. Its reactivity can, in practice, be tested by studying the response of the blood level of extrinsic activator to a standardized stimulation. Most frequently used in this respect is the venous occlusion test. In this test, one of the arms is cuffed for 15 or 20 minutes midway between diastolic and systolic blood pressure (6). A standardized injection of DDAVP (1-desamine-8-D-arginine vasopressin) has been recently introduced as a promising alternative (7).

Intrinsic plasminogen activators

The intrinsic plasminogen activators do not occur as such in the blood but circulate as inactive precursors: plasminogen proactivators. The total amount of activator activity that can be obtained from these proactivators is around 100 $BAU.ml^{-1}$ of plasma, as also shown in Figure 2. The blood level of proactivators does not react to the stimuli for the extrinsic system discussed above (Figure 2). Whether these stimuli can also lead to proactivator activation is not known at present.

The total potential activator activity of $\pm$ 100 $BAU.ml^{-1}$ is due to more than one intrinsic proactivator; various pathways exist for the activation of proactivators. The structure of these pathways and their relations are not fully elucidated yet. A present hypothesis (8) concerning the intrinsic proactivators and their activation is outlined in Figure 3 and discussed below.

ACTIVATION OF PROACTIVATORS

A part of the plasminogen proactivator potential can become activated by a mechanism involving coagulation Factor XII. In this pathway of activation, prekallikrein and high molecular weight kininogen are participants. Studies with factor XII- or prekallikrein-deficient plasmas indicate that the factor XII-dependent pathway accounts for activation of $\pm$ 50% of the total proactivator potential.

The other half appears to be activated by other mechanisms, tentatively designated as factor XII-independent. Consequently, there seems to be at least two pathways of proactivator activation, as indicated in Figure 3.

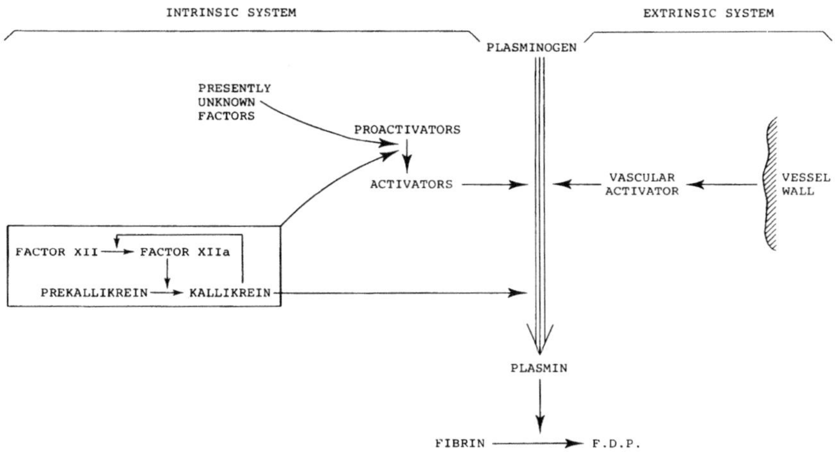

FIG. 3. Scheme for activation of plasminogen-mediated fibrinolysis.

By purification and separation experiments (8), division of the intrinsic activator activity into three fractions can at present be demonstrated (cf Fig. 4). Two of these fractions appear to be activated by the factor XII-dependent pathway.

One of them is identified as being due to plasma kallikrein, an enzyme which contributes 10-15 $BAU.ml^{-1}$ to the total intrinsic activator activity (8).

The other factor XII-dependent activator activity contributes 30-40 $BAU.ml^{-1}$, but still needs further characterization to be certain about its identity. The third portion, contributing 40-50 $BAU.ml^{-1}$ of plasma, appears to be activated independently of factor XII; this activity also needs further biochemical characterization.

Consequently, the available data indicate the occurrence of two different intrinsic proactivator systems involving different pathways of activation and different proactivators as summarized in Figure 4. It should be clear that the above concept is incomplete and much remains to be explored.

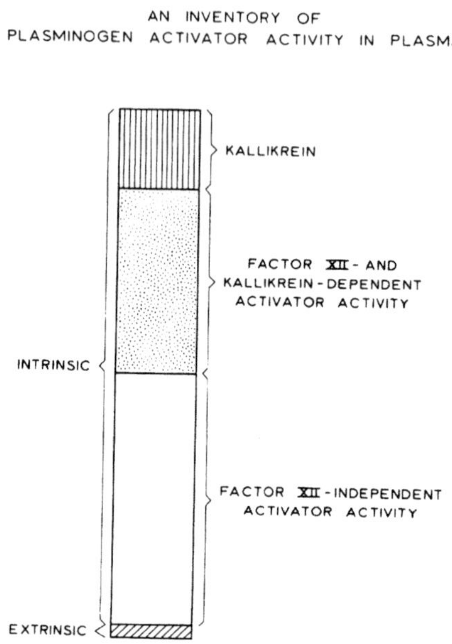

FIG. 4. Quantitative inventory of plasminogen activator activities of plasma. The total column represents 100 $BAU.ml^{-1}$ of normal morning plasma.

The physiological importance of the intrinsic systems has also not yet been studied. We need to be cautious here, since the intrinsic plasminogen activators have so far been investigated only in vitro. It is possible that, in our in vitro assay systems certain enzymes activate plasminogen, while they are not significantly involved in this activation in vivo. For plasma kallikrein we need to consider this possibility seriously, since this enzyme has a very low specific activity for plasminogen (10^4 times lower than urokinase and human tissue activator) and only contributes in vitro due to its relatively high plasma concentration. We have to reckon, however, with all of the above mentioned contributions to fibrinolysis when we measure fibrinolysis in the laboratory. This makes the study of blood fibrinolysis highly complicated.

METHODS FOR MEASURING BLOOD FIBRINOLYTIC ACTIVITY

Traditional methods

Traditional methods for studying the fibrinolytic activity of blood are the dilute blood clot lysis time method and the euglobulin methods.

In the dilute blood clot lysis time method, whole blood is diluted and clotted (9). The lysis time of the clot represents the fibrinolytic activity of the blood. The blood is diluted for the practical reason that clots formed from diluted blood lyse more quickly, presumably because of a relative decrease in fibrinolytic inhibition on dilution.

In euglobulin methods, the fibrinolytic activity of a fraction of plasma is studied (9). In the euglobulin fraction, the fibrinolytically active components of plasma are separated to a large extent from the antifibrinolytic components by isoelectric precipitation. Euglobulin fractions always show a measurable fibrinolytic activity because of this removal of the majority of the inhibitors, whereas the activity in plasma is nearly always completely suppressed by them. The fibrinolytic activity of the euglobulin fraction can be represented by the lysis time of the euglobulin clot (formed by clotting of the fibrinogen present in the fraction) or by the size of lysis zones in a fibrin plate (10).

The fibrinolytic activity observed by these methods originates from extrinsic activator in the blood but also to a certain extent from intrinsic plasminogen activators (11). The intrinsic activator activity is due to partial activation of the intrinsic proactivator system *in vitro* during the procedures of assay.

The traditional methods give indications of variations in the plasma level of extrinsic activator and have been accordingly used for numerous studies. The activation of intrinsic proactivators is, however, variable and furthermore dependent on variations in the extrinsic activator level (11), rendering the methods suitable only for general impressions and large effects.

The need for methods specific for the various plasminogen activation processes is obvious. Such methods may greatly improve diagnosis in plasma fibrinolysis. It is not surprising that application of the traditional methods in clinical practice has not evoked much enthusiasm for studies of plasma fibrinolysis in the past.

Recent methods

Recent methods for studying plasma plasminogen activators and proactivators include methods for measuring plasma kallikrein, the C1-inactivator-resistant activator activity and the blood activator inventory test.

Plasma prekallikrein contributes to in vitro plasminogen activation. Its variations can be recorded easily, since, as a result of the introduction of synthetic chromogenic substrates, assay of plasma kallikrein has been considerably simplified (see refs 12 and 13).

The C1-inactivator-resistant activator test (11) allows the specific and quantitative assay of extrinsic activator activity in plasma. In this test, use has been made of our observation that addition of an excess of C1-inactivator specifically abolishes the intrinsic activator contribution to the euglobulin activity. This enables specific studies on the plasma level of extrinsic activator, including small variations. That C1-inactivator-resistant activity represents extrinsic activator activity indeed is endorsed by the quenching of this activity by antibodies against human tissue-vascular activator (14). The test has made possible the presentation of the behaviour of the extrinsic activator plasma level as in Figure 2.

The blood activator inventory test (15) measures the total amount of activator activity (extrinsic plus intrinsic proactivators) in plasma. In this test, plasminogen proactivators are completely converted to activators. The total amount measured in pooled normal plasma is arbitrarily set at 100 $BAU.ml^{-1}$ and is reasonably stable among healthy persons. At rest, the contribution of extrinsic activator is negligible (cf Figure 2); therefore the test in fact gives the total level of intrinsic proactivators.

The latter two methods are laborious but allow for the first time a more specific and quantitative study on plasma plasminogen activators. Hopefully, additional and easier methods will become available in the near future.

One possibility might be that plasminogen activators can be measured by synthetic chromogenic substrates. The presently available substrates for urokinase and tissue activator, however, lack sensitivity for the low levels of activators (other than kallikrein) in plasma; the level of extrinsic activator at rest is calculated to be $\pm$ 1 ng/ml with an activity comparable to 0.007 IU urokinase per ml plasma; the total activator level of 100 BAU.ml^{-1} is comparable to 0.7 IU.ml^{-1} urokinase activity. Furthermore, specificity faces a great challenge, since plasma contains various other enzymes.

CONCLUDING REMARKS

From the overview on the activation of plasminogen-mediated fibrinolysis presented, it is evident that this system in blood is rather complex. Various routes of activation and various plasminogen activators are involved. Present knowledge concerning this activation, especially with regard to the intrinsic systems, is far from complete. Future research may fill in the gaps and we can hope that the present impression of complexity arises only from our ignorance.

A special problem which has hindered study is the lack of adequate methods to account for the different processes of activation. Improvement of methodology may lead to clinical and fundamental research into the activation systems and their physiological role.

The presence of a powerful system of intrinsic fibrinolysis activation is especially intriguing and has only recently been revealed. It is tempting to speculate that this intrinsic system is of physiological relevance and can be subjected to therapeutic manipulation. It contains a considerable activator potential and recruitement of this potential for thrombolysis may open up a complete new area for fibrinolytic therapy.

REFERENCES

1. Christman JK, Silverstein SC, and Acs G. 1977. Plasminogen activators. In : Proteinases in mammalian cells and tissues, Barrett (Ed), Elsevier, North-Holland Biomedical Press, pp 91-149.
2. Rosing DR, Redwood DR, Brakman P, Astrup T, and Epstein SE. 1973. Impairment of the diurnal fibrinolytic response in man. Effects of aging, type IV hyperlipoproteinaemia, and coronary artery disease. Circ.Res. 32, 752-758.
3. Astrup T. 1977. The physiology of fibrinolysis. In : Thrombosis and urokinase. Proceedings Serono Symposia, Paoletti R and Sherry S (Eds), Academic Press, New York, vol. 9, pp 11-23.
4. Rosing DR, Redwood DR, Brakman P, Astrup T, and Epstein SE. 1978. The fibrinolytic response in man to vasoactive drugs measured in arterial blood. Thromb.Res. 13, 419-428.
5. Alkjaersig N and Fletcher A. 1977. Metabolism of urokinase. In: Thrombosis and urokinase. Proceedings Serono Symposia, Paoletti R and Sherry S (Eds), Academic Press, New York, vol. 9, 129-142.

6. Robertson BR, Pandolfi M, and Nilsson IM. 1972. "Fibrinolytic capacity" in healthy volunteers at different ages as studied by standardized venous occlusion of arms and legs. Acta Med.Scand. 191, 199.
7. Aberg M, Nilsson IM, and Vilhardt H. 1979. The release of fibrinolytic activator and factor VIII after injection of DDAVP. In : Progress in chemical fibrinolysis and thrombolysis, Davidson JF, Cépelâk V, Samama MM, and Desnoyers PC (Eds), Churchill Livingstone, Edinburgh, vol.4, pp 92-97.
8. Kluft C. 1978. Blood fibrinolysis. Proactivators and activators in human plasma. Thesis, Leiden University, The Netherlands.
9. Graeff H and Beller FK. 1971. Fibrinolytic activity in whole blood, dilute blood, and euglobulin in clot lysis time tests. In : Thrombosis and bleeding disorders, Bang NU, Beller FK, Deutsch E, and Mammen EF (Eds), Academic Press, New York, pp 328-331.
10. Haverkate F and Brakman P. 1975. Fibrin plate assay. In : Progress in chemical fibrinolysis and thrombolysis, Davidson JF, Samama MM, and Desnoyers PC (Eds), Raven Press, New York, vol.1, pp 151.
11. Kluft C. 1978. C1-inactivator-resistant fibrinolytic activity in plasma euglobulin fractions : its relation to vascular activator in blood and its role in euglobulin fibrinolysis. Thromb.Res. 13, 135-151.
12. Claeson G, Friberger P, Knös M, and Erikson E. 1978. Methods for determination of prekallikrein in plasma, glandular kallikrein and urokinase. Haemostasis 7, 76-78.
13. Kluft C. 1978. Determination of prekallikrein in human plasma: optimal conditions for activating prekallikrein. J.Lab.Clin.Med. 91, 83-95.
14. Rijken DC. 1980. Plasminogen activator from human tissue. Thesis, Leiden, The Netherlands.
15. Kluft C. 1978. Levels of plasminogen activators in human plasma: new methods to study the intrinsic and extrinsic activators. In: Progress in chemical fibrinolysis and thrombolysis, Davidson JF, Rowan RM, Samama MM, and Desnoyers PC (Eds), Raven Press, New York, vol.3, pp 141-145.

FLUOROGENIC SUBSTRATES AND THE ASSAY OF UROKINASE AND TISSUE PLASMINOGEN ACTIVATOR

G. WIJNGAARDS AND W. NIEUWENHUIZEN
Gaubius Institute, Health Research Organization TNO, Herenstraat 5d, 2313 AD Leiden, The Netherlands.

Synthetic substrates can be used for the assay of various factors of the coagulation and fibrinolytic system. However, synthetic substrates cannot always be used without problems. One of the aspects, emphasized in this chapter, is the sensitivity of synthetic substrate methods. This sensitivity is a function of the efficiency with which a particular substrate is hydrolyzed by the enzyme. When a substrate is degraded with a relatively high efficiency by a particular enzyme as compared with other enzymes, then this substrate is considered to be "specific" for that enzyme. Thus on the one hand the sensitivity problem of a synthetic substrate method is a specificity problem. On the other hand, the sensitivity is also a function of the sensitivity with which the reaction products can be detected. Here we would like to focus on these aspects of the use of synthetic substrates, with special reference to the fibrinolytic system (Fig. 1).

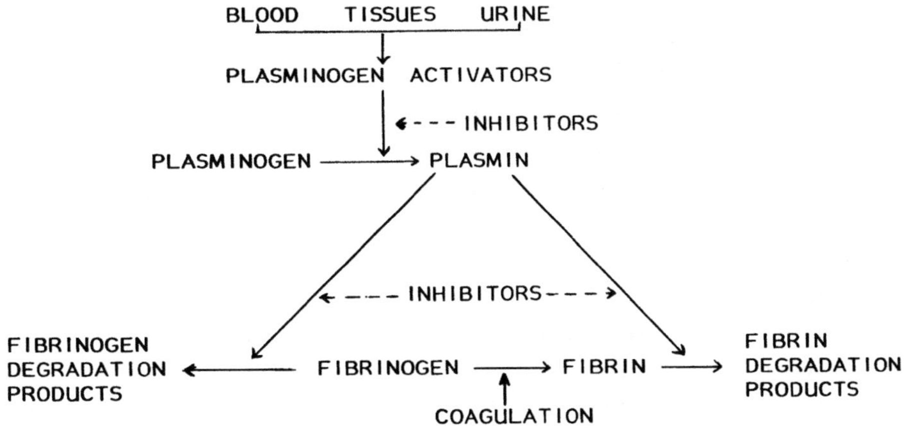

FIG. 1. Schematic representation of the fibrinolytic system.

Traditional assays for measuring the activities of the different fibrinolytic agents are the fibrin plate method, the clot lysis time method, the caseinolytic method and methods based upon these principles with labelled protein substrates. These methods are highly sensitive and rather specific. However, they are not suitable for steady-state kinetic studies and some require long incubation times (e.g. the fibrin plate method). Furthermore, plasminogen activators can be assayed only indirectly via plasminogen activation.

When we started the synthesis of some substrates in early 1976, a rather large number of synthetic substrates was available for the assay of fibrinolytic enzymes, such as α-N-acetyl-glycyl-L-lysine methyl ester (AGLME), α-N-acetyl-L-lysine methyl ester (ALME), α-N-benzoyl-L-arginine ethyl ester (BAEE), α-N-carbobenzoxy-L-lysine p-nitrophenyl ester (CLN), L-lysine methyl ester (LME), α-N-methyl α-N-tosyl-L-lysine β-naphtol ester (MTLNE), α-N-tosyl-L-arginine methyl ester (TAME), and α-N-acetyl-L-lysine-p-nitroanilide (ALNA).

These substrates have a well-defined structure and most of them are suitable for steady-state kinetic studies often in continuous measurements. The specificity and sensitivity of methods based on these substrates, however, are low. With the amino acid esters for instance the esterolytic activities of the enzymes are measured and these may differ from the proteolytic activities. Moreover, biologic fluids often contain esterases and these could contribute to the hydrolysis of the substrates. With the amino acid amides these specificity problems have been overcome to a great extent.

In 1976 the substrates S-2251 (Kabi, Mölndal, Sweden) and Chromozym UK (Pentapharm, Basel, Switzerland) became available. One important difference from the earlier substrates is that the amino acid has been replaced by a tripeptide. This idea of synthesizing a small peptide in order to improve the specificity was first presented in 1972 by Blombäck and coworkers (1). They suggested a sequence similar to the natural substrate as the amino acid sequence of the peptide. This concept was employed in the development of S-2251 and Chromozym UK and has been applied now to the design of various substrates. If this principle were to be applied to develop a substrate for plasminogen activators, the peptide would be pro-gly-arg, since plasminogen activators activate plasminogen by splitting the arginine -valine bound in the amino acid sequence -pro-gly-arg-val- (2). However, synthesis of a substrate consisting of the tripeptide pro-gly-arg with the N-terminal proline blocked and the p-nitroanilide group at the C-terminal side, resulted in a substrate which was hardly hydrolyzed by urokinase (Bergström, personal communication). Now, we know that there is a strong bend in this part of the plasminogen molecule and this probably explains the above observation.

In our attempts to develop a synthetic substrate for plasminogen activators we tried a substrate with the dipeptide gly-arg and two substrates with the tripeptide val-gly-arg. Important in our approach is the choice of a fluorophore as the leaving group in order to increase the sensitivity of the assay.

Several fluorophors could be considered e.g. 7 amino-4-methylcoumarine, 5-aminoisophtalic acid dimethyl ester, 2-naphthylamine and 4-methoxy-2-naphthylamine. Only the latter two are non-fluorescent when bound to the peptide and fluorescent after release by the enzyme. This is an advantage for the sensitivity of the assay because one can work at optimum wavelengths for excitation and emission. In our substrates we used the 2-naphthylamide group.

Figure 2 shows the formulae of the different substrates which we synthesized and tested for their usefulness as substrates for the assay of plasminogen activators.

The results of the degradation of these substrates by urokinase and tissue plasminogen activator are shown in table 1. To obtain some information on the specificity of the substrates we measured also the degradation by human plasmin.

From the comparison of the catalytic efficiencies (k_{cat}/K_m) it can be deduced that these substrates are rather specific for urokinase as compared with plasmin. None of them, however, exhibits excellent kinetic parameters. The most striking observation was that tissue activator from the human uterus could only split substrate II (5,6). Substrates I and III (with a free amino terminus) were not hydrolyzed by this activator at a measurable rate. This strongly suggests that

TABLE 1.

Kinetic parameters of the hydrolysis of some fluorogenic substrates by plasmin, urokinase, and tissue plasminogen activator (3,4)

Parameter	PLASMIN			UROKINASE			TISSUE ACTIVATOR		
	I	II	III	I	II	III	I	II	III
pH Optimum	8.2	7.5	8.0	8.5	8.0	8.8	–[a]	8.5	–[a]
K_m apparent (mmol/liter)	1.7	1.6	0.9	7.5	1.1	0.6	–[a]	0.5	–[a]
V_{max}[b]	0.6	2.4	1.2	21.8	3.0	4.8	–[a]	2.4	–[a]
Specific activity (U/mg)	0.019	0.078	0.039	2.9	0.4	0.6	–[a]	N.D.[c]	–[a]
k_{cat} (sec^{-1})	0.03	0.11	0.05	3.6	0.5	0.8	–[a]	N.D.[c]	–[a]
k_{cat}/K_m (liter/sec mmol)	0.02	0.07	0.06	0.48	0.45	1.33	–[a]	N.D.[c]	–[a]

[a] No detectable hydrolysis.

[b] For plasmin, in nanomoles per CU per minute, and for urokinase and tissue activator, in picomoles per CTA unit per minute.

[c] N.D. = not determined.

I = glycyl-L-arginine-2-naphthylamide.
II = t-BOC-L-valyl-glycyl-L-arginine-2-naphthylamide.
III = L-valyl-glycyl-L-arginine-2-naphthylamide.

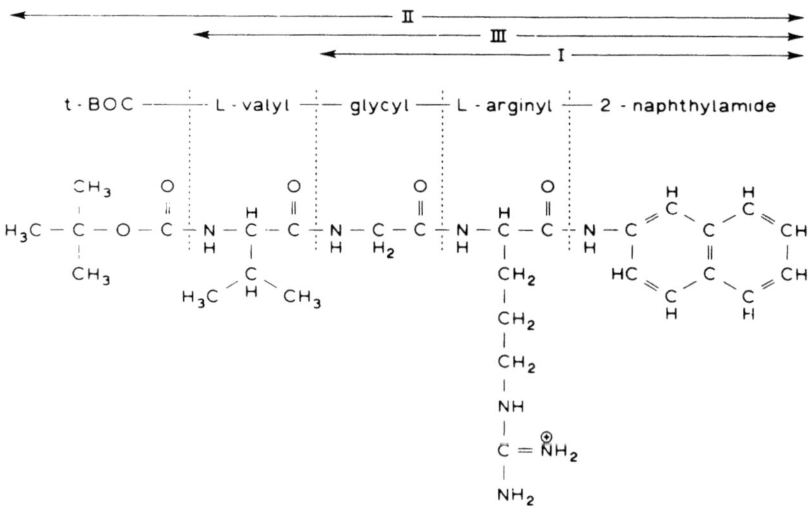

FIG. 2. Fluorogenic plasminogen activator substrates (3,4)

a blocked amino terminus is an essential substrate requirement for tissue activator.

A reflection of these differences between urokinase and tissue plasminogen activator is found in some newly developed substrates by KABI (viz. S-2227 and S-2444) (Table 2).

TABLE 2.
Activities of urokinase and tissue plasminogen activator on some recent synthetic substrates from KABI (6).

Substrate	Formula	Activity* (ΔA/min) of Urokinase	Tissue plg act
S-2227	L-glu-gly-L-arg-pNA	0.16	0.04
S-2444	L-pyroglu-gly-L-arg-pNA	0.24	0.16
S-2322	D-val-gly-L-arg-pNA	0.14	0.15

* The fibrinolytic activities of urokinase and tissue plasminogen activator (as determined by the bovine fibrin plate method) were chosen equal (90 IU/ml, final concentration).

Although the fibrinolytic activities of the urokinase and tissue plasminogen activator preparations are equal, their rates of hydrolysis of substrate S-2227 differ considerably. This difference is greatly diminished by internal blockade of the amino-group of the aminoterminal glutamic acid residue via cyclization to the pyroglutamyl group (L-pyroglu) thus yielding substrate S-2444. An interesting feature is exhibited by substrate S-2322. This substrate does not have a blocked amino terminus but the amino-terminal valine is in the D- instead of the L-configuration. Urokinase and tissue activator have equal activities on this substrate.

The results obtained with S-2227 and S-2444 confirm our earlier conclusions that an essential substrate requirement for tissue plasminogen activator is the presence of a blocked amino-terminal amino acid. However, the results with S-2322 demonstrate that this conclusion does not apply to a D-amino acid. The use of combinations of S-2227 and S-2444, of S-2227 and S-2322 or of our substrates I (or III) and II may allow the discrimination and assay of urokinase and tissue plasminogen activator activities.

Although the specificity of the substrates has been greatly improved at present, the problem of the insufficiently low detection limit of the leaving groups still remains. Some investigators (7,8) have tried to overcome this problem by performing a secondary chemical reaction to obtain a modified reaction product with a higher molar extinction coefficient.

A secondary chemical reaction, however, can be harmful to the enzyme(s) under investigation and therefore a direct quantification of the leaving groups is preferable. In this respect fluorogenic substrates offer a solution. This can also be deduced from several other investigations on the development of fluorogenic substrates for fibrinolytic enzymes. Clavin et al. (9) and Bigbee et al. (10) synthesized peptides linked with a 4-methoxy-2-naphthylamine group. Pochron et al. (11) prepared a peptide with a 5-amino-isophthalic acid dimethyl ester, while Pierzchala et al. (12), Iwanaga et al. (13) and Morita et al. (14) used 7-amino-4-methylcoumarine (MCA) as the fluorophor. In general, the sensitivity of the assays with these substrates is improved as compared with chromogenic substrates, but the maximum profit expected from the use of fluorometry is not obtained. This is due to the relatively poor kinetic properties of the fluorogenic substrates studied thus far.

Interestingly, from the work of Morita (14) it can be concluded that plasmin is unable to split the arg-MCA bond.

Summarizing, all the observations mentioned thus far demonstrate that the specificity and sensitivity of a particular substrate for a particular fibrinolytic enzyme are determined by four parameters :

a) the amino acid sequence of the peptidyl part;
b) the presence or absence of a blocked L-amino terminus. Also the structure of the group attached to the amino-terminus seems to influence the kinetic properties (Kluft, personal communication);
c) the configuration of the amino-terminal amino acid (D or L);
d) the nature of the group linked with the carboxy terminal amino acid.

Drapier et al. (15) incubated a plasminogen activator together with plasminogen and a plasmin substrate (S-2251) and followed the increase in optical density versus time. For the mathematical treatment of the results they derived a simple formula from which the activator activity can be calculated, provided that the K_m and k_{cat} of the hydrolysis of S-2251 by plasmin are known (see figure 3 and formulae). This is achieved by simply plotting the concentration of product formed against the square of the reaction time (t^2). This plot gives a straight line (Figure 3, right panel) of which the slope is directly proportional to the amount of activator present in the assay system. This type of assay is specific by definition as long as a specific substrate for plasmin is used. Furthermore, a multiplication factor is introduced by the small cascade process and thus the sensitivity is increased. Since S-2251 is a rather specific substrate for plasmin, the method of Drapier et al. (15) can be used without noticeable snags. Probably its sensitivity can be greatly improved by using a specific fluorogenic instead of a chromogenic substrate for plasmin. Although the principle of the Drapier-method is attractive it must be realized that sufficient quantities of a defined plasminogen (glu- or lys-plasminogen) must be available and that plasmin inhibitors, such as α_2-antiplasmin, must be absent from the assay medium.

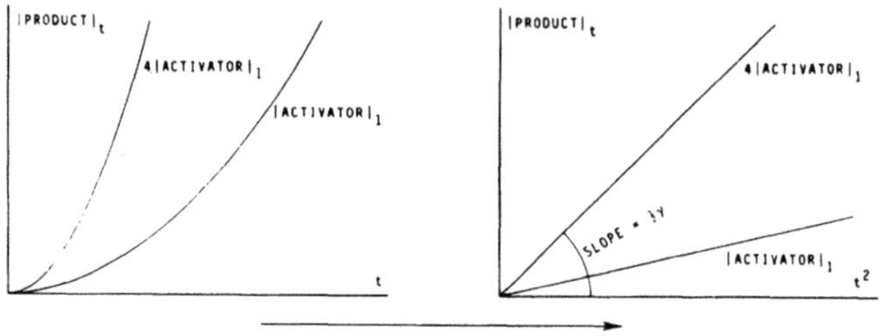

$$\text{PLASMINOGEN} + \text{ACTIVATOR} \underset{Km_1}{\rightleftharpoons} (\text{PLASMINOGEN} \,.\, \text{ACTIVATOR}) \xrightarrow[k_1]{} \text{PLASMIN} + \text{ACTIVATOR}$$

$$\text{PLASMIN} + \text{SUBSTRATE} \underset{Km_2}{\rightleftharpoons} (\text{PLASMIN} \,.\, \text{SUBSTRATE}) \xrightarrow[k_2]{} \text{PLASMIN} + \text{PRODUCT}$$

if $|\text{SUBSTRATE}| \gg Km_2$ and $|\text{PLASMINOGEN}| \approx \text{CONSTANT}$

then: $|\text{PRODUCT}|_t = \frac{1}{2}\gamma t^2 + v_o t + |\text{PRODUCT}|_o$

where $\gamma = \dfrac{k_1 k_2 |\text{ACTIVATOR}|}{1 + \dfrac{Km_1}{|\text{PLASMINOGEN}|}}$

v_o = PLASMINOGEN-INDEPENDENT RATE OF HYDROLYSIS

$|\text{PRODUCT}|_o$ = CONCENTRATION OF PRODUCT AT $t = o$

FIG. 3. Principle of the plasminogen activator assay according to Drapier et al. (15).

REFERENCES

1. Svendsen L, Blombäck B, Blombäck M, and Olson PI. 1972. Synthetic chromogenic substrates for determination of trypsin, thrombin and thrombin-like enzymes. Thromb.Res. 1, 267-278.
2. Wiman B and Wallén P. 1975. Amino acid sequence around the arginyl-valyl bond in plasminogen which is cleaved during the second step of the activation process. Thromb.Res. 7, 239-243.
3. Nieuwenhuizen W, Wijngaards G, and Groeneveld E. 1977. Fluorogenic peptide amide substrates for the estimation of plasminogen activators and plasmin. Anal.Biochem. 83, 143-148.
4. Nieuwenhuizen W, Wijngaards G, and Groeneveld E. 1977. Synthetic substrates and the discrimination between urokinase and tissue plasminogen activator activity. Thromb.Res. 11, 87-89.
5. Rijken DC, Wijngaards G, Zaal-de Jong M, and Welbergen J. 1979. Purification and partial characterization of plasminogen activator from human uterine tissue. Biochim.Biophys.Acta 580, 140-153.
6. Rijken DC. 1980. Plasminogen activators from human tissue. Thesis, Leiden, The Netherlands, p. 70.
7. Kwaan HC, Friedman RB, and Szczecinski M. 1978. Amplification of color yield of chromogenic substrates using p-dimethylaminocinnamaldehyde. Thromb.Res. 13, 5-13.
8. Green GJD and Shaw E. 1979. Thiobenzyl benzyloxycarbonyl-L-lysinate, substrate for a sensitive colorimetric assay for trypsin-like enzymes. Anal.Biochem. 93, 223-226.

9. Clavin SA, Bobbitt JL, Shuman RT, and Smithwick EL Jr. 1977. Use of peptidyl-4-methoxy-2-naphthylamides to assay plasmin. Anal.Biochem. 80, 355-365.
10. Bigbee WL, Weintraub HB, and Jensen RH. 1978. Sensitive fluorescence assays for urokinase using synthetic peptide 4-methoxy-β-naphthylamide substrates. Anal.Biochem. 88, 114-122.
11. Pochron SP, Mitchell GA, Albareda I, Huseby RM, and Gargiulo RJ. 1978. A fluorescent substrate assay for plasminogen. Thromb. Res. 13, 733-739.
12. Pierzchala PA, Dorn CP, and Zimmerman M. 1979. A new fluorogenic substrate for plasmin. Biochem.J. 183, 555-559.
13. Iwanaga S, Kato H, Maruyama I, Adachi N, Ohno Y, Takada K, Kimura T, and Sakakibara S. 1979. Fluorogenic peptide substrates for proteases in blood coagulation, kallikrein-kinin and fibrinolysis systems : substrate for plasmin and factor XI_a. Thrombos. Haemostas. 42, 49.
14. Morita T, Kato H, Iwanaga S, Takada K, Kimura T, and Sakakibara S. 1977. New fluorogenic substrates for α-thrombin, factor X_a, kallikreins, and urokinase. J.Biochem. (Tokyo) 82, 1495-1498.
15. Drapier JC, Tenu JP, Lemaire G, and Petit JF. 1979. Regulation of plasminogen activator secretion in mouse peritoneal macrophages. I. Role of serum studied by a new spectrophotometric assay for plasminogen activators. Biochimie 61, 463-471.

DISCUSSION

R. Lijnen : In the absence of fibrin isn't this plasminogen activator a very poor activator? Can you use this method in a plasma system?

G. Wijngaards : This is indeed a problem related to the "Drapier" assay. A difference between fibrinolytic assays and this assay is that fibrin is absent. From several studies we know that fibrin seems to behave as an important cofactor in the activity of tissue and other plasminogen activator preparations, while it is not for urokinase. However, fibrin is not suitable in spectrophotometric assays because of its insolubility. This problem has to be solved. Allen and Pepper developed a method for the preparation of soluble fibrin polymers. These soluble fibrin polymers can function, like fibrin, as a cofactor and could be used in a spectrophotometric assay. Another possibility is the use of the more-defined poly-lysine; it seems that this has a similar effect on plasminogen activators as fibrin and soluble fibrin polymers.

GENERAL DISCUSSION AND CONCLUSIONS

GENERAL DISCUSSION AND CONCLUSIONS

D. Collen : At the conclusion of this meeting, I think we should discuss some of the advantages and problems related to assays with chromogenic substrates and the indications for their possible application to routine hemostasis analyses. One practical question is whether the present synthetic substrates are specific enough for the assays that have been discussed today?

H.C. Hemker : As a rule they are specific enough. When the method is well designed few complications arise because of aspecificity.

G. Wijngaards : This is valid for the situation in the coagulation field, but in fibrinolysis specificity is still a problem for most of the individual enzymes. Only for prekallikrein is the sensitivity high enough, for plasmin the specificity is rather good, but there is still a need for substrates with improved specificity for the activators and enzymes involved in the activation of plasminogen.

D. Collen : Is there any indication that the source of the enzymes used to measure inhibitors (being factor Xa for heparin assay, thrombin for AT III assay, plasmin for antiplasmin assay) is important for the results?

L.H. Kahlé : Concerning the antithrombin assay I can say that one year ago I did a comparison between bovine and human thrombin in the assay system; with human thrombin the affinity e.g. the inhibition was somewhat higher. But if you express the result in the conventional way, in a percentage of normal pool plasma, then you see no difference in the values.

D. Collen : Different types of thrombin (e.g. α- or γ-thrombin) have different clotting and amidolytic activities. Does this influence measurements of thrombin or antithrombin III with chromogenic substrates?

H.C. Hemker : It doesn't matter in all the tests where thrombin is freshly generated from prothrombin, but it may matter when you are comparing different thrombin preparations that have been stored for various periods of time.

P. Friberger : We have stored different thrombin solutions for weeks and months in the refrigerator. Thrombin stored in the refrigerator for one or two months will degenerate into β- or γ-thrombin, but we stil got exactly the same inhibition by plasma using these preparations.

D. Collen : Did you still obtain the same amidolytic activity per unit of thrombin?

P. Friberger : Yes, we did in most cases. And even if we get decreased activity on a substrate, we obtain the same slope for the standard curve. Our experiments also show that thrombin that is not active on the substrate does not consume any antithrombin.

D. Collen : How do coagulation and synthetic substrate assays for the same parameter compare? I think we have concluded that for AT III and presumably also for the heparin assays the correlation is quite good. But for the anticoagulant control at the present time there are significant discrepancies and problems.

L.H. Kahlé : When in future comparisons are made, the system should be well described, because, as we saw, if you use RVV from a different source you get different results. Sometimes you can of course have good correlation, but you want the same absolute value, and if you want a standardization you need a good definition. I think at the moment most assays are not well described relating to pH, buffer, ionic strength, ...

H.C. Hemker : I could not agree more. Most systems reported in the literature are so badly described that it is hard to repeat them.

D. Collen : How is the comparison of data obtained with chromogenic and fluorogenic substrates?

G. Wijngaards : It is difficult to compare the data because the leaving group of the fluorogenic substrates is different from that of the chromogenic substrates and this group influences the kinetic parameters of the substrates. When the only difference between substrates is the presence of a chromogenic instead of a fluorogenic leaving group, we find different kinetic data. In general, the kinetic data are less favourable for the fluorogenic substrates, usually the K_m values are higher and V_{max} values lower.

Another aspect related to this comparison is the equipment that you use; especially for the fluorometric methods the quality of the equipment is important for the sensitivity. Roughly one can say that fluorometric methods are from 10 to 100 or 500 times more sensitive than chromogenic methods, depending on the quality of the equipment.

H.R. Lijnen : These fluorescent measurements are strongly influenced by quenching in solution. Can you dilute plasma enough to avoid this quenching and still have the high sensitivity to measure for instance very low concentrations of plasminogen activator?

G. Wijngaards : Scattering is a major problem you have to be aware of. Therefore we pass buffer and substrate solutions through a millipore filter to eliminate all dust in order to obtain a stable baseline. Then the high sensitivity of the method can be optimally utilized and allows such strong dilution of plasma that the quenching you refer to is no longer a problem.

D. Collen : How do the different chromogenic substrates for the same type of assay compare to each other?

R.M. Bertina : For the factor II assay we have compared S-2238 and the chromozym TH and they gave identical results. Only the chromozym TH has a higher cross-reaction with bovine Xa and S-2238 has a higher cross-reaction with human Xa. So, you have to use different activators in the assay, dependent on the actual substrate used.

H.C. Hemker : I had the same comment.

D. Collen : What is the cost to benefit ratio from the point of view of a large laboratory with a high turnover and of a small laboratory with only a few determinations a day? How does this compare with other methods, i.e. prothrombin times?

H.C. Hemker : Reduced work is not the only benefit. If it becomes possible to have automated assays for the factors II, VII and X in anticoagulated patients then we may be able to define much better the therapeutic range of these factors so that we can apply better anticoagulation.

Unidentified discussant : I don't know about the benefit but if you have to buy factor deficient plasma and you compare with a factor

II or X assay then factor II by chromogenic assay costs 40 cents and by clotting assay about 3 gulden. For factor X chromogenic it is 1 gulden where the clotting test costs about 3 gulden; the chromogenic substrates are thus not that expensive.

D. Collen : The prothrombin time test for the control of anticoagulant therapy is very cheap. That will be hard to beat.

Unidentified discussant : We determine clotting factors by chromogenic assay when the prothrombin time is prolonged, and we can do it now for less than half the price.

H.C. Hemker : I would like to ask the manufacturers if these substrates would still stay that expensive when they become more generally used. People making polypeptides told me that polypeptides cost about 1 gulden per gram, per amino acid.

P. Friberger : When production is on a larger scale, prices may go down. However, I am not responsible for the prices, so this is just my private opinion.

D. Collen : May I conclude that eventually the cost of a chromogenic assay will most probably not be prohibitive?

The applications for chromogenic substrates that were discussed today are : 1) anticoagulant control; 2) diagnosis of severe liver disease; 3) diagnosis of vitamin K deficiency; 4) AT III determination; 5) heparin assay; 6) α_2-antiplasmin assay; and 7) measurement of plasminogen activators in biological fluids. I would like to suggest that we review these indications and try to make some recommendations.

With respect to the indications for anticoagulant control, it appears that more work has to be done to develop these assays for routine application. There are two main problems : the correlation between the chromogenic assays and prothrombin time and secondly the present determinations of factor X and II may not be as useful in the beginning of anticoagulant therapy. Do we agree that it is at present too early to bring these assays into clinical practice?

With respect to the monitoring of liver function it appears that factor X, AT III, α_2-antiplasmin and probably factor II are decreased in liver disease. Does this have any pathophysiological meaning and are there therapeutical implications? Should we advise physicians to perform any of these tests in a significant number of patients with liver disease or only in exceptional cases with bleeding complications?

J.W. ten Cate : If you want us to make a choice, I would advise the cheapest and most reliable method at the moment. I don't know the prices of all the clinical chemistry methods, but AT III could add more information than i.e. albumin.

D. Collen : So, in the present state these tests should not be part of a liver function analysis on a routine base.

Dr. Bertina has presented a combined assay with 2 methods of activation to measure vitamin K deficiency. Are there any comments on this method?

H.C. Hemker : I think it is a good method, but it will not give any more information than a classical clotting test.

D. Collen : Dr. Bertina has said that these assays are more sensitive to detect low grade vitamin K deficiency. With additional work there might be an additional application : is that correct?

R.M. Bertina : Apart from being more specific they prove directly that there is vitamin K deficiency, where the clotting tests always have to be checked for other possibilities, i.e. low factor VII concentrations due to other causes.

H.C. Hemker : As I already said, I should like to see this confirmed in the same series of patients.

D. Collen : Several speakers have said today that AT III determinations may have definitive indications. I understood that it should not be a general screening method for conditions such as venous thrombosis or in postoperative patients, but it could add valuable information in patients with DIC, toxemia and also possibly in the nephrotic syndrome with extensive proteinuria. Something else?

J.W. ten Cate : I came to the same list; nephrotic syndrome because in the case of AT III deficiency you have to treat these patients with heparin or prophylactically with oral anticoagulants; thrombosis of unknown origin in young people, certainly if there is a positive family history; DIC in general, to evaluate the mechanism, because it is not necessarily always thrombin; bleeding problems particularly in liver cirrhosis and possibly in toxemia.

L. Wijnja : The AT III determination by chromogenic substrate is routinely used in our general hospital. In my opinion this is useful for our patients in the field of internal medicine, surgery and gynecology. So, I advise the AT III tests in general practice.

D. Collen : What are the indications for performing a heparin assay? Dr. Holm suggested that heparin therapy should be monitored strictly to keep a patient's blood level above 0.3 U/ml and below 0.7 U/ml, at least for therapeutic heparin doses.

H.A. Holm : Yes, I agree. What we have shown is that this assay is useful in monitoring heparin therapy, but we have also seen that other conventional methods may be useful. So, it is more or less a practical problem.

D. Collen : Do you think there is any indication to measure low heparin levels in subcutaneous prophylaxis?

H.A. Holm : As a general rule I would not recommend this, but it is a very good method to have when a patient on low-dose heparin is bleeding.

D. Collen : With respect to the fibrinolytic inhibitor α_2-antiplasmin Dr. Samama indicated that at the present stage this assay is mainly useful for research applications and maybe for monitoring thrombolytic therapy. Apart from the investigation of a bleeding tendency of unknown origin which may be due to an extremely rare congenital deficiency of α_2-antiplasmin there appears to be no real indication for the routine performance of the α_2-antiplasmin assay.

M. Samama : Except maybe in compensated DIC.

D. Collen : The last application of chromogenic substrate assays which has been discussed today is the determination of fibrinolytic activators At present these methods can however not be applied to biological fluids as such.

G. Wijngaards : That is correct. The latest development by Drapier has still to be tested for biological materials. But it seems very attractive since plasminogen is incorporated in the system thus increasing the specificity.

D. Collen : May I conclude this discussion with the statement that at the present time two assays using chromogenic substrates have routine applicability, namely AT III and heparin assays, both in selected conditions. The control of anticoagulant therapy has to be postponed until more research has been done. I would like to thank all the speakers and participants on behalf of the Organizing Committee of this symposium for their interest and collaboration.

GPSR Compliance

The European Union's (EU) General Product Safety Regulation (GPSR) is a set of rules that requires consumer products to be safe and our obligations to ensure this.

If you have any concerns about our products, you can contact us on ProductSafety@springernature.com

In case Publisher is established outside the EU, the EU authorized representative is:

Springer Nature Customer Service Center GmbH
Europaplatz 3
69115 Heidelberg, Germany

Batch number: 10607224

Printed by Printforce, the Netherlands